中英双语版

THE CHARM OF TRADITIONAL CHINESE MEDICINE I

神奇的中医药

（一）

赵继荣 米登海 / 主编

武永胜 郭亚银 师育兰 / 译

Chief Editors: Zhao Jirong   Mi Denghai

Translators: Wu Yongsheng   Guo Yayin   Shi Yulan

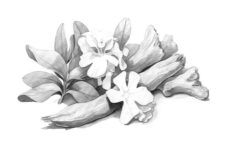

甘肃科学技术出版社

Gansu Science and Technology Press

甘肃·兰州
Lanzhou, Gansu

图书在版编目（CIP）数据

神奇的中医药. 一：汉、英 / 赵继荣，米登海主编；
武永胜，郭亚银，师育兰译. -- 兰州：甘肃科学技术出
版社，2024.9. -- ISBN 978-7-5424-3216-2

Ⅰ.R2-49

中国国家版本馆CIP数据核字第2024B858Y1号

神奇的中医药（一）（中英双语版）

SHENQI DE ZHONGYIYAO (YI) (ZHONG-YING SHUANGYU BAN)

赵继荣　米登海　主编

武永胜　郭亚银　师育兰　译

项目策划	朱黎明　杨丽丽
翻译策划	刘　唱　张艳萍　舒　畅
译文主审	郭亚银　武永胜
责任编辑	于佳丽
封面设计	石　璞

出　版　甘肃科学技术出版社

社　址　兰州市读者大道568号　　730030

电　话　0931-2131575（编辑部）　　0931-8773237（发行部）

发　行　甘肃科学技术出版社　　印　刷　甘肃兴业印务有限公司

开　本　787毫米×1092毫米 1/16　印　张　8.75　插　页　1　字　数　126千

版　次　2024年9月第1版

印　次　2024年9月第1次印刷

印　数　1~2300

书　号　ISBN　978-7-5424-3216-2　　　　定　价　68.00元

出　版　说　明

　　中医药学包含着中华民族几千年的健康养生理念及其实践经验,是中华文明的一个瑰宝,凝聚着中国人民和中华民族的博大智慧。学习中医药文化,可以补充医学知识,培养健康养生理念,启发科学探索,亦可促进国际文化交流。因此,我们策划并出版中医药文化科普图书《神奇的中医药(中英双语版)》系列,以便高校、科研院所的国际交流生、在华生活的外籍人员乃至大众了解中医药文化的渊源和本真。

　　本丛书专为普及中医药文化而作,以提纲挈领的方式,向读者介绍中医药文化的精髓。第一、二册循序渐进,各有侧重。第一册讲述:中医药学的起源与发展、中医药学故事、古今中医药学教育、中医药学对世界的贡献,旨在帮助读者了解中医药学的发展脉络;第二册则涵盖:走近中医药、中医药学蕴藏的智慧、中药与方剂、甘肃中医药故事及生活中的中医保健;旨在帮助读者了解中医药学的理论体系、追溯中医药文化的根源。每本书通过 25 个经典、有趣的故事,将中医药文化娓娓道来。本丛书内容精炼,图文并茂,兼具科学性、通俗性和趣味性。

　　甘肃是中医药文化重要的发祥地之一,在中医药学教育方面也有着深厚的国际交流积淀。作为资深的中医药学者、践行者兼教授,本书作者以系统的思维、清晰的逻辑,深入浅出地向读者介绍中医药及其文化的精髓。在编写和出版过程中,我们进行了深层次的研究和探索,广泛征求意见,反复修改,精益求精,但可能依旧存在疏漏与不足之处,恳请各位老师、同学指正。希冀这套书不断优化,成为中医药文化的优秀双语科普读物,为人们了解中医药文化提供便捷。

PUBLICATION NOTES

Traditional Chinese Medicine (TCM) encompasses the health-preserving philosophy and practical experience of the Chinese nation spanning thousands of years. It is a treasure of Chinese civilization and embodies the accumulated and profound wisdom of the Chinese nation. Studying TCM culture can broaden medical knowledge, foster wellness concepts, inspire scientific exploration, and facilitate cultural exchanges between nations. Therefore, we have planned and published *The Charm of Traditional Chinese Medicine* (*Chinese-English Edition*), a series of popular science books on TCM culture, which is intended to introduce the origin and essence of TCM to international exchange students in Chinese universities and research institutes, foreigners living in China, and the public at large.

This two-book series is specifically designed to popularize TCM culture, presenting the readers with the quintessence of TCM culture in a concise and comprehensive manner. With each book having its own focus, the chapters are gradually and progressively arranged. The first covers the origin and development of TCM, stories or legends about TCM, ancient and modern TCM education, and the contributions of TCM to the world, aiming to make the readers fully informed about the evolutions of TCM. The second contains an introduction to TCM, great wisdom embedded in TCM, numerous medicines and formulas, stories about particular physicians or medicines in Gansu, and TCM healthcare in daily life, aiming to help the readers understand the theoretical system of TCM and the context of TCM culture. Moreover, each book is adequately illustrated with colour pictures and skillfully interspersed with 25 classic and amusing stories or anecdotes about TCM culture. All this makes the books concise and informative as well as readable and absorbing.

Gansu, one of the important birthplaces of TCM culture, boasts considerable experience of international exchange in TCM education. As seasoned scholars, practitioners and professors of TCM, the authors have employed a systematic and logic approach to make a general and popular introduction of the essence of TCM and its culture to the readers. Throughout the compilation and publication of the books, we editors and translators have conducted thorough research and exploration, canvassed diverse opinions, and made repeated revisions, and strived for perfection. However, there may still be omissions, deficiencies or errors, and we kindly ask our readers to point them out. We hope that this series will be improved and finally become an excellent bilingual popular science publication on TCM culture, providing convenience for people interested in TCM culture.

目 录
Contents

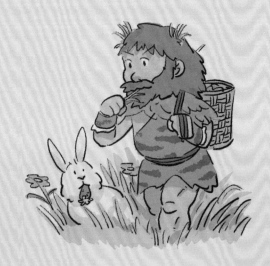

第一单元　中医药学的起源

中华民族是世界上历史最悠久的民族之一，远在6万多年前，在黄河流域的甘肃省天水市秦安县诞生了大地湾文化，之后不断迁徙融合，发展壮大。而中医药学是中华民族生生不息、繁衍不止的重要保障。

中医药学的起源非常早，早在远古时期，当时的人们食草根树皮来充饥，慢慢了解了一些草本植物的功效。随着生产技术的提高，人们开始打磨工具，逐渐出现了砭（biān）石和骨针，也就是针灸针具的雏形。人们发现用其刺激身体某些部位有止痛等功效。火的发明，出现了灸、熨烫等疗法，大大缓解了人们的痛苦。

Unit I   Origins of Traditional Chinese Medicine

The Chinese nation is one of the oldest in the world. More than 60,000 years ago, the Dadiwan culture was born in Qin'an, Tianshui, Gansu Province, in the Yellow River Basin. And after that, the Chinese culture grew, migrated, merged, developed and expanded continuously. And Traditional Chinese Medicine (TCM) provided an indispensable guarantee for the Chinese people to thrive and multiply.

TCM originated from very ancient times when people fed on grass roots and bark and gradually understood the medical efficacy of some plants. With the improvement on production skills, people began to polish stones into tools, and gradually invented stone and bone needles, which were the embryonic forms of acupuncture needles, it was found that pain could be more or less relieved by stimulating or piercing some parts of the body with those stone and bone needles. And with the invention of fire therapies of moxibustion and ironing appeared, which greatly alleviated people's pain.

　　后来，神农尝百草，慢慢获知了很多药物的用途，商朝的伊尹(yī yǐn)又发明了把草药熬煮成汤服用的方法，减轻了生吃药物的危害。到了东汉时期，《黄帝内经》《神农本草经》《伤寒杂病论》等著作的问世，标志着中医药学体系的建立。所以说，中医药学是世界上历史最悠久的医学，是我们中华民族的骄傲。

Later, legend has it that Shennong, the Divine Farmer, tasted many wild plants and gradually learned about their medical efficacy. Yi Yin of the Shang dynasty invented decoction to reduce the harm of eating raw herbs. In the Eastern Han dynasty (AD 25-220), the publication of *Huangdi Neijing* (*Huangdi's Classic of Medicine*), *Shennong Bencao Jing* (*Shennong's Herbal*) and *Shanghan Zabing Lun* (*Treatise on Exogenous Febrile and Miscellaneous Diseases*) marked the establishment of the system of TCM. Therefore, TCM, one of the oldest medicines in the world, is the pride of the Chinese nation.

第一章　钻木取火与中医药

在数十万年前的远古时期,我们的祖先在与大自然的搏斗中学会了使用钻木取火的方法获得火种,祖先们用火照明、驱吓夜间偷袭的野兽,用火驱散了洞穴中的寒冷与潮湿,更重要的是用火加热食物,消灭了生肉中的寄生虫,减少了由于生吃食物而引起的疾病,从而提升了体质,延长了寿命。

在使用火的过程中,人们发现在用火烤制食物时,难免被火灼伤皮肤,可能偶尔发现,某个部位皮肤被灼(zhuó)伤,反而会减轻消除某些病痛,这种经验日积月累,人们便有意识地点燃某种植物茎叶,来灼烤身体的某些部位以治疗疾病。有时候烤火取暖,在刚烧过火的石头上睡觉,那热乎乎的石头,挨着疼痛的腰腿部位,让疼痛减轻了很多,慢慢地,灸法、热熨(yùn)法就被发现了。

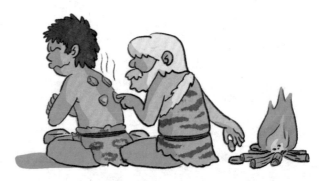

Chapter 1 Drilling Wood to Make Fire and Traditional Chinese Medicine

In the primitive times hundreds of thousands of years ago, our ancestors learned how to drill wood to make fire in their struggle with difficulties in nature. Fire was used to illuminate, frighten wild animals that attacked them at night and get rid of the cold and damp in the caves where they lived. More importantly, they made fire to heat food and eliminate parasites in raw meat, which reduced diseases caused by eating raw food, thereby improving their physical constitution and prolonging their life span.

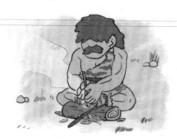

In the process of using fire, people would be inevitably burned by fire while roasting food, and occasionally they found that this would relieve pain or even eliminate some diseases, if a certain part of the skin was burned. With the accumulation of such experience, people consciously lit the stems and leaves of some plants to scorch some parts of the body to cure themselves of certain diseases. Sometimes they slept on the heated stones on which a fire had been kept for warmth, and felt the pain on the waist and leg having been relieved a lot. Slowly, moxibustion and the therapy with hot compresses were thus discovered.

第二章　神农尝百草

在远古时期，人们不懂医药知识，不知道植物可以用来治疗疾病，大家得了病只能硬扛着，身体健壮的年轻人遇见一些不严重的疾病尚能硬挺过去，但是老年人和小孩常会因为疾病而死亡。当时有个部落的首领叫神农，看着百姓被疾病折磨非常痛心，便决心为大家找寻治病的办法。

有一天，神农偶尔尝了田野里的杂草，发现草木有酸甜苦辣等味道。他就将带有苦味的草，给咳嗽不止的人吃，吃完后，咳嗽症状立刻减轻不少；把带有酸味的草，给肚子疼的人吃，这个人的肚子就不疼了。于是神农发现了药草可以为人类治病。

Chapter 2 Shennong Tasted Herbs

In the antiquity, people knew nothing about medicine or about the fact that plants could be used to treat diseases. When they were stricken with a sickness, they had only to endure it. Only strong young people could survive some minor diseases, while old people and children often died of these diseases. At that time, Shennong, a tribal leader, was very sad to see his people suffering from diseases, and was determined to find a cure for them.

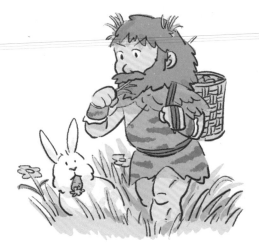

One day, Shennong by chance ate some weeds in the fields and found that the plants tasted sour, sweet, bitter or spicy. He let the people who suffer from persistent cough eat some bitter grass, and the coughing were immediately much alleviated; he let the people who had a stomachache eat some sour grass and the stomach soon stopped hurting. That was how Shennong discovered that some herbs could be used to treat human diseases.

后来,神农又品尝了很多草本植物,了解了它们的不同功效,总结出能治病的药物越来越多。可是神农尝百草是十分辛苦的事,不仅要跋山涉水寻找草木,而且品尝草药还有生命危险。有一次,他品尝一种开小黄花的植物,刚把花和茎吃了之后,就感到肚子钻心地痛,好像肠子断裂了一样,痛得他满地打滚。最后神农没有能挺住,被这种草所毒死。神农虽然被毒死,却用他的生命发现了一种含有剧毒的草——断肠草。

这便是神农为民尝百草的传说,后来,人们为了纪念神农,便将他封为"炎帝",尊为"三皇五帝"之一,而把中华儿女称之为"炎黄子孙"。中国第一部药物学专著就叫《神农本草经》。

Thereafter, Shennong tasted more wild herbs and learned about their different medical efficacy, concluding that more plants could be used to treat various diseases. It was a very hard task for Shennong to taste all kinds of herbs, because he had not only to trek in the mountains and cross rivers to find wild plants for medicinal purposes, but also risked his life to taste herbs. Once he tasted a plant with small yellow flowers, and as soon as he had taken in the flowers and stems, he felt a sharp pain in his stomach, as if his intestines were broken, making him roll all over the ground. In the end, Shennong ended up being poisoned by the plant. That was the manner in which he died, but his sacrifice of his own life helped identify a highly poisonous grass, *duanchangcao* (Gelsemium elegans).

Thus goes the legend of Shennong tasting hundreds of wild herbs for the people. Later on, in order to commemorate him, people named him "Emperor Yan", respected him as one of the "great rulers in ancient China". And thus the Chinese people call themselves "descendants of Emperors Yan and Huang". The first book on pharmacology in China was called *Shennong Bencao Jing* (*Shennong's Herbal*).

《神农本草经》古籍
An Ancient Version of the *Shennong Bencao Jing* (*Shennong's Herbal*)

第三章　汤药的由来

今天，中医大夫治病，开的中药方剂很多都是将中药材熬煮在一起的药汤，那大家知道，为什么中药要熬成药汤才能服用？

在原始社会，人们起初发现药草能治病后，都是直接把药放在嘴里嚼服，结果，由于药材没有加工，肠胃不好消化，影响了治疗效果，而有的药物是有毒的，直接吃下去就会危及生命。比如我们前面说到的神农，就是生服了断肠草而去世的。

Chapter 3 The Origins of Decoction

Today, when they treat diseases, doctors of Traditional Chinese Medicine (TCM) make up prescriptions and boil some Chinese medical herbs together to make decoctions (liquid medicines). Do you know why Chinese herbal medicines must be boiled into decoctions before they are taken?

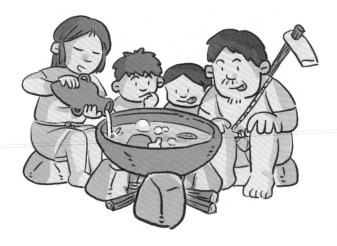

In primitive society, when people first discovered that herbs could cure diseases, they chewed and swallowed them. But herbs were not easy to digest before being processed, which would affect their therapeutic effects. Some herbs, if eaten directly were poisonous and would endanger people's lives. For example, Shennong, who we mentioned above, died of *duanchangcao* (Gelsemium elegans).

　　后来，人们有了陶器，可以把食物煮熟。到了商朝时期，有位著名的丞相叫伊尹，伊尹原是商汤妻子陪嫁的奴隶，他聪慧灵敏、精明能干，精通烹饪，还懂得医药知识，因此能够成为商朝的丞相。伊尹根据烹调方法，将桂枝、芍药、甘草、生姜、大枣这些食物佐料熬煮，用于疾病的预防和治疗，在当时对药物功效和毒性尚未深入了解的条件下，这些汤药既能减少直接服用药物容易中毒的危险，还能起到治病和保健的作用。后来，伊尹又教会大家用陶罐把不同的草药配合，加水熬煮成汤服用，既安全，效果还好。他还研究出了很多汤药方，因此后世尊称他为汤药之祖。

Chapter 4 Bianque and the Secret of *Guasha*

The *guasha* (scrapping therapy) is often shown on TV. But who invented this treatment? The answer is Bianque, a famous doctor in the Spring and Autumn period.

Bianque, a doctor living over 2500 years ago, was proficient in many forms of treatment of TCM. According to the *Shiji* (*Records of the Grand Historian*), Bianque was passing through the State of Guo and heard that its prince had died and a funeral was being held in the palace. He asked the people about the prince's disease, and learned that the prince was suddenly out of breath when frightened. Bianque suspected that the prince might not actually be dead. So he requested permission to go into the palace to observe the prince's appearance, and claimed that he could make the prince come back to life, but everyone was quite surprised to hear this!

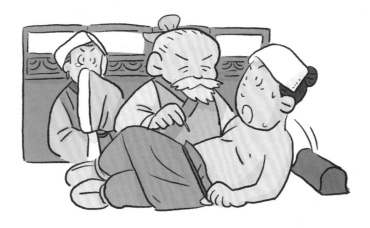

扁鹊给太子把过脉后，确认他只是一时休克而已。于是扁鹊快速地在太子的头、胸、足的几个穴位施针治疗，果然不一会儿太子就苏醒了，之后太子继续服用了扁鹊的汤药，很快就康复了。这件事被大家广为流传，世人都说扁鹊是起死回生的神医。

这里所说的施针，就是用砭（biān）石磨制的针，而这里的施针主要是指用砭石针按压，刺激，或较浅地刺入肌肤。除了施针，扁鹊还给太子整个背部进行刮痧，引导气血运行，这里所用的刮痧板就是砭石制作的。

由于扁鹊高超的医术，今天人们在形容某位医生医术高明的时候就会说他"扁鹊再世"。

After feeling the prince's pulse, Bianque confirmed that he was only in a coma. Bianque gave needle acupuncture therapy in the prince's head, chest and feet. Sure, after a while the prince regained consciousness. After taking Bianque's decoction, he soon recovered. The story was widely circulated, and therefore Bianque was said to be a miracle doctor who could make the dead come alive!

The needle mentioned in the story is one ground with stone, and the therapy mentioned in the story mainly refers to one with stone needles being used to press, stimulate, or shallowly penetrate the skin for treatment. In addition to needling, Bianque also scraped the whole back of the prince to promote the circulation of qi and blood. And the guasha board used in the process was made of stone.

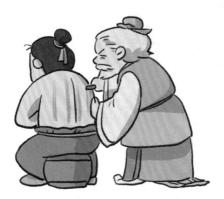

Because of Bianque's excellent medical skills, people today would describe such a doctor as Bianque.

第五章　伏羲创制八卦的传说

伏羲(xī)、女娲是中华民族的始祖。他们的传说,在中国代代相传、家喻户晓。相传,甘肃天水为伏羲与女娲的出生地,直到今天,这里仍在每年举行盛大的公祭伏羲活动,以纪念这位"中医药之祖"。

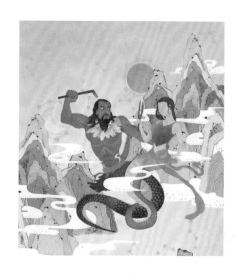

伏羲带领人们用兽皮缝制衣服,抵御寒冷,而狩猎活动的展开又使得动物类食物日益增加,很大程度上增强了百姓适应自然环境的能力。他带领人们围着篝火跳舞,以驱寒取暖,强健身体,却发现通过这种运动,可以祛除身上的一些病痛,这便是传统体育活动及导引术的雏形。他还观天文、察地理,通晓日月阴阳的道理,始创了八卦,成为中医学思想的主要文化根源之一。至今,天水市还有相传伏羲创制八卦的卦台山。

Chapter 5 The Legend of Fuxi Creating the Eight Trigrams

Fuxi and Nuwa were the ancestors of the Chinese nation and the legends about them have been passed down from generation to generation in China and are well known to all. It is said that the present Tianshui, Gansu Province is the birthplace of Fuxi and Nuwa, where a grand public ceremony for Fuxi is still held annually to commemorate this "ancestor of Traditional Chinese Medicine (TCM)".

Fuxi led people to sew animal skins into clothes to resist the cold, and people learned to hunt and increased foods from animals day by day, which greatly enhanced their ability to adapt to the natural environment. He also led people to dance around the open fire to keep warm and strong, and found that some pains and diseases could be relieved or removed by such exercises, which were regarded as the embryonic form of traditional Chinese sports and the Mawangdui daoyinshu (a regimen in the ancient times which combines breathing exercises and body movement). He also observed celestial bodies and geographical features tried, to understand the law of the sun and the moon, and established eight trigrams, which became one of the main cultural roots of TCM. It was said that Fuxi created the eight trigrams on the Guatai Mountain, located in Tianshui.

　　"八卦"不是一种具体器物的发明，而是一个哲学思想的萌芽，是华夏文明取之不竭的智慧源泉。德国数学家莱布尼茨研究八卦，从"两仪、四象、八卦"中得到启发而发明了二进位制，现在广泛地应用于生物及电子学中。

The "eight trigrams" is not the invention of a concrete utensil, but the germination of a philosophical thought and an inexhaustible source of wisdom of Chinese civilization. German mathematician Leibniz studied the eight diagrams, and inspired by the "two elementary forms, four emblematic symbols, eight trigrams", he invented the binary system, which is now widely used in biology and electronics.

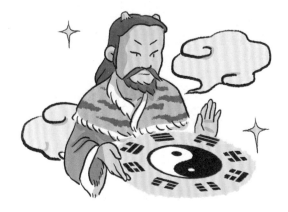

第二单元　中医药学的发展

经过人们长时间医学经验的积累总结,到了秦汉时期,中医药学确立了下来,各个学科逐渐有了专门的典籍。

后来经过历朝历代的发展,中医药理论和临床实践越来越丰富,出现了很多著名的医学家,在更多的研究领域获得了更为丰富的成果。

这样一脉相承、绵延数千年一直未曾中断的医药文化及文明,是世界医学史上所罕见的。中国古典医籍数量之大,名医辈出,人数之多,在同时期的世界范围内也不多见。中国传统医药学有着强有力的生命力,它随着时代的前进而发展。经过了与近代医药文化的撞击、对抗到结合,也从国外先进文化中吸取有用的东西,出现了中西医结合的探索,传统医学逐渐走向现代化。

Unit II Development of Traditional Chinese Medicine

Through a long period of accumulation of medical experience, Traditional Chinese Medicine (TCM) was established in the Qin and Han dynasties, and various subjects gradually developed and their respective canons were written and published.

With the going on of successive dynasties, the theories and clinical practices of TCM became more and more abundant, and many figures emerged as famous medical experts, making more and greater achievements in more research fields.

TCM, together with its relevant culture, has lasted for thousands of years without interruption, which is a phenomenon quite uncommon in the history of medicine across the world. It is also uncommon that, during the same period of history, there had been so many doctors hailed as the best in their days and many medical classics were written by them. TCM has been developing with much vitality and always kept pace with times. After its collision, confrontation and combination with modern Western medicine and its culture, TCM has been trying to take in anything useful from advanced foreign cultures, and to explore ways of integrating itself with western medicine. Therefore, TCM is moving towards its own modernization.

第六章　张仲景与《伤寒杂病论》

在中医学几千年的历史中,涌现出了非常多的名医大家,张仲景无疑是其中的佼佼者。

张仲景的父亲曾经做过官,因此他从小就读了许多书,学问非常好。他的父亲本来想让他当官,可是张仲景所处的时代正是动荡的东汉末年,连年混战,人民深受苦难,饥寒困顿,各地连续暴发瘟疫,很多人都病死了。看到这样的情况,使得张仲景下定决心成为一名可以救死扶伤的医生。

为了学习医术,张仲景去拜当时的名医张伯祖,张伯祖见他聪明好学,又有刻苦钻研的精神,就把自己的医学知识毫无保留地传授给他,后来张仲景尽得其传,且青出于蓝而胜于蓝。

Chapter 6 Zhang Zhongjing and the *Treatise on Exogenous Febrile and Miscellaneous Diseases*

In the history of thousands of years of Traditional Chinese Medicine (TCM), many famous doctors appeared, among whom Zhang Zhongjing was undoubtedly one of the best.

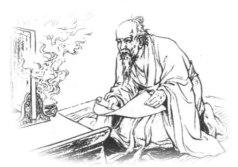

His father being an official, Zhang Zhongjing, could afford to read many books since childhood and became knowledgeable. At first his father wanted him to be an official too, but in the turbulent Late Eastern Han dynasty in which Zhang Zhongjing lived, people suffered incessantly from continuous war, hunger and cold, and many people died of successive outbreaks of plague. Seeing that, Zhang Zhongjing made up his mind to become a doctor who could save people's lives.

In order to learn medicine, Zhang Zhongjing went to visit Zhang Bozu, a famous doctor at that time. Zhang Bozu found that Zhongjing was smart, eager to learn and studious, so he unreservedly imparted his medical knowledge to him. Later, Zhang Zhongjing learned all that his teacher could teach him and surpassed his teacher in medicine.

作为一名医生，张仲景认真吸收当时人们同疾病做斗争的丰富经验，结合个人临床诊治疾病的丰富经验和心得体会，创造性地著成了《伤寒杂病论》这一部划时代的医学巨著，使得中医学理论与临床紧密结合起来，奠定了中医学辨证论治的治疗原则。

《伤寒杂病论》是中国医学史上影响最大的著作之一，在其成书后近2000年的时间里，一直指导着中医学的发展，被公认为是中国医学方书的鼻祖。书中的很多知识至今仍在临床广泛应用。因此，张仲景被尊称为中华民族的"医圣"。

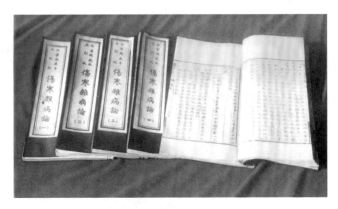

《伤寒杂病论》古籍
An Ancient Version of the *Shanghan Zabing Lun*
(*Treatise on Exogenous Febrile and Miscellaneous Diseases*)

As a doctor, Zhang Zhongjing earnestly fed himself with others' rich experience in fighting against diseases, combined his own studiously gained clinical experience, and creatively wrote the *Shanghan Zabing Lun* (*Treatise on Exogenous Febrile and Miscellaneous Diseases*), which closely combined the theory of TCM with its clinical practice and laid a foundation for the principle of syndrome differentiation and treatment in TCM. So the classic was seen as a major landmark in the development of TCM.

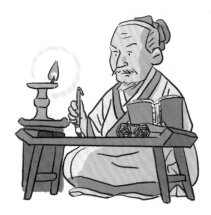

The *Shanghan Zabing Lun*, as one of the most influential works in the history of TCM, has been guiding the development of TCM for nearly 2000 years since its completion, and is recognized as the originator of medical books of its own kind in TCM. Much of the knowledge in this work is still widely used in clinical practice. Therefore, Zhang Zhongjing has been honored as the "medical sage" of the Chinese nation.

第七章　华佗与五禽戏

民间有很多关于神医华佗的故事和传说。在《三国演义》中，他为东吴大将周泰治枪伤，为关云长"刮骨疗毒"，为曹操医治"头风"病而被害等故事家喻户晓，妇孺皆知。

华佗是三国时期的著名医生，当时天下大乱，疫病流行，老百姓苦不堪言，华佗就决心做一名良医，为百姓解除痛苦。他刻苦学习医学，仔细阅读历代名医的医书并加以发展。他的医术十分高明，不管什么疑难杂症，到了他手里大都药到病除，特别擅长外科手术，他是首个在手术中使用麻醉药的人。

Chapter 7 Hua Tuo and the Wuqinxi

There are many stories and folklore about the miracle doctor Hua Tuo. In the novel *The Romance of the Three Kingdoms*, some stories about Hua Tuo are very well-known, for example, he treated the spear wounds of General Zhou Tai, a general of Eastern Wu State, cured General Guan Yu of the arrow poison by scraping the bones, and he was killed unfortunately for treating the "head wind" disease of Cao Cao.

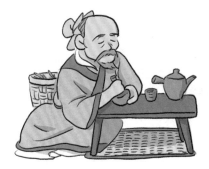

Hua Tuo was a famous doctor in the Three Kingdoms period when the country was in a chaos, with epidemics prevalent, and the common people were unspeakably miserable. Hua Tuo was determined to be a good doctor to relieve the sufferings of the common people. He assiduously studied medicine, carefully read the medical books by famous doctors of the past periods and improved on them. He attained such a high level of expertise in medicine that he could cure most of the serious complicated diseases, and he was especially highly skilled at surgery, being the first Chinese doctor to use anesthetics during surgery.

很早以前人们就发现一些药物具有让人昏睡的功效,华佗把这些药物配制成"麻沸散"。在外科手术之前叫病人服下这个药,等到麻醉药效发挥功用后就替病人做手术。在1700多年前能做这种全身麻醉的大手术,是相当了不起的事,所以人们称他为"神医"。

华佗不仅医术高明,还注重健身养生,为世人创编了一套模仿五种禽兽姿态的健身操——五禽戏。

五禽戏,是模仿虎、鹿、熊、猿、鸟5种动物的神态与动作而编创的一套健身运动。人们模仿这些姿态,可以锻炼筋骨、畅通气血,达到祛病防疾、益寿延年的目的。

据传,华佗的学生吴普施行这种方法锻炼,活到90多岁时,仍耳聪目明,牙齿也完整牢固。

A long time ago, people found that some herbs had the effect of making people sleepy, and Hua Tuo concocted them in *mafeisan,* a prescription that could anaesthetize patients before an operation. When *mafeisan* had taken effect on a patient, Hua Tuo performed the operation. More than 1700 years ago, it was really a great achievement that he was able to perform operations under general anesthesia, so people called him a "miracle doctor".

Hua Tuo not only was excellent at medical skills, but also paid attention to fitness and health care. He created a set of fitness movements, the wuqinxi (five-animal boxing), which imitated the maneuvers of five kinds of animals.

The wuqinxi is a set of fitness exercises in imitation of the expressions and movements of tigers, deer, bears, apes and birds. By imitating these postures, people can exercise their muscles and bones, regulate the circulation of the qi and blood, for the purpose of preventing diseases and prolonging their lives.

Legend has it that Hua Tuo's student Wu Pu practiced the wuqinxi, and in his 90s, he still had good hearing, eyesight, and strong teeth.

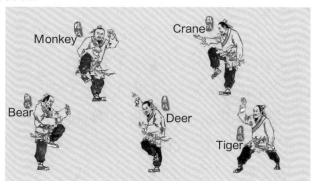

五禽戏动作示意图
Schematic Diagram of the Wuqinxi
(In the above pictures, people are doing the movements that imtate the motion of the bear, monkey, deer, crane and tiger.)

第八章　"针灸鼻祖"皇甫谧

皇甫(fǔ)谧(mì)相传是甘肃灵台人,从小就寄养在叔父家。小时候,他不爱劳动,也不爱学习,特别贪玩,直到20岁还成天东游西逛,无所事事,他的叔叔和婶婶见他这个样子,深为他的前程感到担忧。

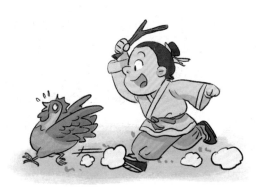

有一次,皇甫谧到瓜市上去玩,有个卖瓜的人给了他一个瓜,皇甫谧很有孝心,把瓜送给了婶婶。谁知婶婶仍然不高兴地说:"你不知道学习,我心里最不安了。你送什么给我吃,我也不高兴!"说罢,她长长地叹了一口气。婶婶接着开导他说:"先前孟子的母亲为了孟子学好,三次搬家;曾子用杀猪的办法教子;我虽然比不上他们,但也够苦口婆心的了。你怎么一句也听不进去?你什么时候才能知道用功学习呢?"说着,婶婶伤心地哭了起来。婶婶的耐心教育,最终感动了皇甫谧。他想:孟子能成为有用的人,为什么我就不能?他当即向婶婶表示:今后再也不贪玩了,抓紧时间学习,做个有用的人。

Chapter 8 Huangfu Mi, the Originator of Acupuncture and Moxibustion

Legend has it that Huangfu Mi hailed from Lingtai, Gansu Province, and was fostered in his uncle's home from an early age. When a child, he was too much of a good-time boy to do any serious studying and working. Before he was 20 years old, he had spent all his days idling about the neighborhood, and, seeing him behaving like that, his uncle and aunt were very worried about his future.

Once when Huangfu Mi hanged around a market, a melon seller gave him a melon out of filial affection for his uncle and aunt, he gave the melon to his aunt. But she was still unhappy with him and said, "You don't like reading, and I feel most worried. Whatever you give me can't make me happy!" And after a long sigh, she went on to have an enlightening talk with him, "In the past, Mencius'mother moved their home three times so that Mencius could get a better environment for studies. Zengzi taught his son by killing a pig. Although I am not as persuasive as them, I have tried my best to educate you. Why have you been so deaf to my words? When will you want to study hard? "No sooner had she finished than she began to cry sadly. Auntie's earnest persuasion finally touched the heart of Huangfu Mi. He thought, "Now that Mencius could become a useful person, why can't I?" He immediately said to his aunt, "I will never play again. I will cherish the time to study and become a useful person."

从此以后,皇甫谧拜有学问的席坦为师,努力学习,并且变得勤快了:他常常帮助叔叔到田里干活,帮助婶婶干家务事。这样日复一日,年复一年,学业大有长进,品德也为乡人所敬仰。皇甫谧后来得了病,行动不便,给他的学习带来困难。可是,他还以坚韧不拔的毅力,孜孜不倦地学习。别人劝他注意身体,他却说:"我早晨学到了知识,就是到晚上死了也心甘情愿。"

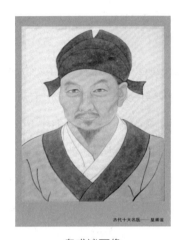

皇甫谧画像
Portrait of Huangfu Mi

皇甫谧把古代著名的三部医学著作,即《素问》《针经》《明堂》集合起来,并结合自己的亲身经验,编纂成一部针灸学巨著——《针灸甲乙经》,这是中国现存最早的一部理论联系实际,有重大价值的针灸学专著,一向被列为学医必读的古典医书之一,对针灸学以至整个中医学事业的发展作出了巨大的贡献。由此他被人们尊称为"中医针灸学鼻祖"。

From then on, Huangfu Mi took the learned Xi Tan as his teacher, studied hard and became diligent: he often helped his uncle work in the fields and his aunt do housework. In this way, day after day, year after year, he made great progress in his studies, and his virtue was also admired by the villagers. Huangfu Mi later fell ill and became mobility-impaired, which made it difficult for him to study. Yet he studied tirelessly with perseverance. Others advised him to pay attention to his health, but he replied,"I would gladly have learned knowledge in the morning and died at night."

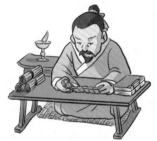

Based on his own clinical experience and three famous ancient medical works: *Suwen* (*Basic Questions*), *Zhen Jing* (*Classic on Acupuncture*) and *Ming Tang* (*a book on acupuncture and moxibustion*), Huangfu Mi compiled a masterpiece on acupuncture and moxibustion: *Zhenjiu Jiayi Jing* (*A-B Classic of Acupuncture and Moxibustion*), as the earliest extant monograph on acupuncture and moxibustion, with high value, the book has made a great contribution to the development of acupuncture and moxibustion as well as the whole TCM and ranks as one must-read medical classic. Therefore, Huangfu Mi was honored as "the originator of acupuncture and moxibustion".

第九章　葛洪与葛根

　　葛洪是中国著名的化学家和医药学家,葛洪带领弟子工作的时候,因为房间里都是烟,时间长了,两个徒弟出现了口臭牙痛、大便不通,身上出现很多红疹的症状,看到这种情况,葛洪很是着急。一天他翻阅医书,发现一种生在山谷中的青藤,根像白玉菇,渣像麻,榨出的汁略带甘甜,喝了可以清热解毒,可以治疗这些疾病。

　　第二天一大早,葛洪独自一人上山寻找这种草药,在一处松软的黄土坡边,葛洪发现了一株粗壮的青藤,用棍撬(qiào)松硬土,将藤根挖了出来,在山泉里洗掉了藤根上的泥土,扛着青藤回来了。葛洪将青藤根切成片状,用锤子敲烂,挤出里边的白浆,煮熟了给两个弟子饮用。喝下浆水,两个弟子便感到燥热的身体逐渐舒适了下来,没几天,病就全好了。

Chapter 9 Ge Hong and *Gegen*

Ge Hong was a famous chemist and herbalist in ancient China. Once, when guiding his students to work, he found two of them suffered from halitosis, toothache and constipation as well as red rash on the body after working for a long time in the room full of smoke. Seeing that, Ge Hong was very anxious. One day while browsing through a medical book, he came upon a kind of green vine usually growing in a valley, whose root, the book said, was like a white jade mushroom, and whose dregs were like hemp. Its pulp, slightly sweet, had the function of clearing heat evil, removing toxin and could cure the above-mentioned diseases.

Early the next morning, Ge Hong went up the mountain alone to look for this herb. On the edge of a soft loess slope, he found a green stout-stemmed vine. He used a stick to pry open the hard soil around it, dug out the roots, washed off their dirt in a mountain spring, and carried them back home. Ge Hong cut the root of the vine into slices, smashed them with a hammer, squeezed out the white pulp inside, and cooked them for the two students to drink. After taking in the cooked pulp, the two felt their heated bodies gradually became comfortable, and in a few days, their illness was completely cured.

　　青藤能解毒治病的消息一传十，十传百，当地百姓纷纷按葛洪的指点，挖青藤根来清热解毒，渐渐的，人们发现这青藤不仅能治病，还能当粮食充饥。青藤锤烂后能和麻一样，可以织布制衣。于是就并大量采种繁育，一时间传遍大江南北。当时，青藤还没有名字，众人只知是葛洪发现传扬开来的，于是就将这青藤取名为"葛"，葛的根自然就被称为"葛根"了。

　　葛洪的医学著作是《肘后备急方》，中国第一位诺贝尔生理学或医学奖获得者屠呦呦就是从这本书里发现了青蒿素的提取线索，从而发明了治疗疟疾的特效药——青蒿素。

The news that the vine could detoxify the body and cure diseases spread like a wildfire. Local people then dug vine roots to detoxify themselves under the instruction of Ge Hong. Gradually, people found that the vine could not only cure diseases, but also serve as food source to relieve hunger. When hammered into hemp, the bark of the vine could be used to weave into clothes. Therefore, it was for a time a fashion for people to cultivate its seeds across the country. At that time, the green vine was yet nameless, and people only knew that it was discovered by Ge Hong, so they named it "Ge", and the root of Ge was naturally called "*gegen*" (kudzu vine root).

The famous medical book written by Ge Hong is *Zhouhou Beiji Fang* (*Handbook of Prescriptions for Emergencies*), by which Tu Youyou, the first Nobel Prize winner in Physiology or Medicine in China, was inspired to extract *qinghaosu* thus developing a specific drug against malaria, namely, artemisinin.

第十章 发明寸口脉法的王叔和

王叔和是东汉末至西晋年间最著名的名医，曾做过曹操的专职侍医，最后升到太医令，是当时掌管国家医药的最高官职。他学识渊博，非常喜欢钻研，他对中医学的主要贡献是他著述的《脉经》和整理了张仲景的《伤寒杂病论》。

《脉经》是中国现存第一部完整的研究脉学的书籍，前代的医家虽然对脉学研究也有一定的成果，却始终没有能够总结归纳，对于脉象名称、诊脉方法等等都比较混乱。王叔和通过多年的行医经验，对诊脉进行了非常细致的规范，并创立了寸口切脉法，为后世的医家一直沿用至今，所以王叔和在诊脉方法上作出了巨大的贡献。

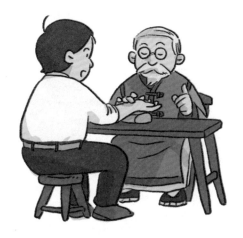

Chapter 10 Wang Shuhe and His Cunkou Pulse-taking

Wang Shuhe was the most famous doctor from the end of the Eastern Han to the Western Jin. He once served as Cao Cao's full-time attending physician, and finally was promoted minister of imperial medical affairs, in charge of national medicine at that time. He was a man of profound learning and liked to study very much. His main contributions to Traditional Chinese Medicine (TCM) were a pulse classic *Mai Jing* (*Pulse Classic*) and the collation of the *Shanghan Zabing Lun* (*Treatise on Exogenous Febrile and Miscellaneous Diseases*) written by Zhang Zhongjing.

The *Mai Jing* was the first complete book on sphygmology in China. Although previous physicians had made some achievements in the study of sphygmology, they had not been able to summarize it, and were confused about the names of pulse manifestations, the methods of pulse diagnosis etc. Through years of medical practice, Wang Shuhe carried out a very detailed regulation of pulse taking, and created the distinctive method of feeling the pulse at the cankou (a location on wrist over the radial artery where pulse is taken), which has been used by later physicians up to now; thus Wang Shuhe made a great contribution to the method of pulse feeling.

切脉在古代是医生了解病情最重要的手段，但是由于是用手来感觉，可能每个人感觉都会有所误差，而这个误差可能就会酿成大祸。所以王叔和在细分脉象时，对相似的脉象如何分辨做了系统的描述。

In ancient times, feeling the pulse was the most important means for doctors to understand the illness, but because it was felt by fingers, sometimes the feeling may not be exact, and an error arising from this might cause misdiagnosis. Therefore, Wang Shuhe made a systematic description as to how to distinguish similar pulse manifestations when subdividing them.

第三单元　中医药学故事

中医的形成、发展都是在厚实的中国传统文化的沉淀中发展起来的。在漫长的历史长河中，名医的故事、中药的传说故事成为中华传统文化的重要组成部分。

黄帝是传说中原各族的共同领袖；岐伯，传说中的医家，黄帝的臣子。现存中国最早的中医理论专著《黄帝内经》就是以黄帝与岐伯讨论医学，并以问答的形式成书的。后世称中医学的"岐黄""岐黄之术"，即源于此。

Unit Ⅲ Stories of Traditional Chinese Medicine

The formation and development of Traditional Chinese Medicine (TCM) are based on an accumulation of Chinese traditional culture. In the long history, the stories of famous doctors and legends on TCM have become a most important part of Chinese traditional culture.

It is said that Huangdi was the common leader of all nationalities in the Central Plain of China, and Qi Bo was a physician as well as a courtier of Huangdi. *Huangdi Neijing* (*Huangdi's Classic on Medicine*), the earliest extant monograph on the theory of TCM in China, was written in the form of questions and answers between Huangdi and Qi Bo. This is the origin of "Qi Huang" or "Qi Huang Zhi Shu (techniques of Qi Huang)" in TCM.

　　悬壶济世是神医与慈善的合名词,《后汉书·费长房传》载,市中有一老翁卖药,悬一壶于市头。而他的药给人治病,每每药到病除,十分有效,引起人们的注意。结果发现这个神奇的老头,每到落市关门后,他就跳入葫芦里。古代医药不分家,就把"悬壶"作为行医的代称。一些医生也将葫芦作为招牌,表示开业应诊之意,后人称医生的功绩为"悬壶济世"。

　　杏林是中医学界的代称,三国时董奉,医术高明,医德高尚,为人治病,不受谢,不受礼,只要求治愈者在他房前栽杏树作为纪念。数年后他用这些杏子换来的谷子救济贫民。人们非常感谢他,送他的匾额上写"杏林""医林""誉满杏林""杏林春暖"。这些赞誉之词成为医德高尚、医术高明的雅称。

The story of "Xuan Hu Ji Shi" (hanging a gourd to help the world or practice medicine to help people) refers to a miracle doctor of deep sympathy. According to *Houhan Shu Fei Zhang-fang Zhuan* (*The Biography of Fei Zhangfang in the History of the Later Han Dynasty*), there was once an old man who sold medicine in the market. He hung a gourd filled with medicine at his market stand. Every time he treated a patient, his medicine worked so well that people soon noticed him and found that this strange old man would jump into the gourd after the market closed. In ancient times, treatment and pharmacy were not separated, so "hanging the gourd" was used as a sign for practicing medicine. Some doctors who started to practice medicine also use a gourd as a signboard to show he was going for medical practice, and later generations praised the deeds of such physicians as "hanging a gourd to help the world (practice medicine)".

"Xing Lin" is another name refering to medicine in China. During the Three Kingdoms period, Dong Feng, a doctor with excellent medical skills and noble medical ethics, treated people without any charge. Instead, he just asked the cured to plant an apricot tree in front of his house as a souvenir. Years later, he exchanged the apricots from the apricot woods for millet to relieve the poor of hunger. People thanked him very much and sent him a plaque with the words like "Apricot Woods" "Medical Woods" "Apricot Woods with Honors" and "Apricot Woods in Warm Spring". Afterwards all these words of praise have become an elegant name for a doctor with noble medical ethics and excellent medical skills.

苍生大医是对医德高尚之人的代称,唐代药王孙思邈,医德高尚,堪称医学界的典范。他在《千金要方》中写道:"若有疾厄(灾难)来求救者,不得问其贵贱贫富,怨亲善友,华夷智愚,普同一等,皆如至亲之想。不得瞻前顾后,虑吉凶,护惜身命。深心凄怆,勿避昼夜、寒暑、饥渴、疲劳、一心赴救,无作功夫形迹之心,如此可成苍生大医。"后人将医德高尚的医生尊称为"苍生大医"。

A great doctor for the people refers to ones with noble medical ethics, like Sun Simiao, China's king of medicine (an excellent herblist) in the Tang dynasty, who had noble medical ethics and can be regarded as a model in the medical field. He stated in *Qianjin Yao Fang* (*Essential Prescriptions for Emergencies*), "If someone who develops a disease or suffers disaster, cries for help, do not ask if he is noble or humble, rich or poor, a resentful relative and a good friend, a Chinese and a foreigner, wise and foolish, he or she should be treated as a close family member. Do not be overcautious and indecisive, or think too much about your own fortune or misfortune, or try to protect your safety and be afraid of losing your life. With deep sympathy, no matter in day and night, cold and heat, hunger and thirst or fatigue, a doctor should be fully dedicated to saving life, asking for no merit or praise, and in that way can one become a great doctor for the people." Thus later generations honored doctors with noble medical ethics as "great doctors for the people".

第十一章　杏林春暖的传说

当我们走进一些传统文化氛围较浓的中药房时，往往能看到"杏林春暖，橘（jú）井泉香"等醒目佳句，而"杏林"与"橘井"自古以来就是中医药的代名词，那这两个典故又是从何而来呢？

"杏林"的典故来自三国时期，那时候在吴国有一位民间医生名叫董奉，定居于庐山之下，医术高明，热心为人治病。但他有一个奇怪的规矩，就是他治病从来不取分文，只需要栽上几棵杏树就可以了。这样连续过了好多年后，所种的杏树已有十万余棵，郁郁葱葱，蔚然成林。

Chapter 11 The Legend of Spring Warmth in the Apricot Woods

Walking into some Traditional Chinese Medicine (TCM) pharmacies with strong cultural ambience, we can often see striking lines inside of them, such as "Warm Spring in the apricot wood, Fragrance of orange leaves and well water". "Xing Lin (apricot wood)" and "Orange Well" have been synonymous with TCM since ancient times. Where do these two allusions come from?

Legend has it that there was a folk doctor named Dong Feng in the State of Wu during the Three Kingdoms Period, who settled at the foot of the Lushan Mountain. He had excellent medical skills and was enthusiastic about treating sick people. But he set up a strange rule: never take a penny for treating a patient; instead, he would ask his patient to plant a few apricot trees at his place. After many years, more than 100,000 apricot trees had been planted, and thus a lush and green apricot wood came into being.

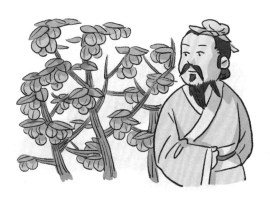

后来,杏子成熟了,董奉就在杏林中搭建了一个谷仓,告诉人们说:"但凡有买杏子的人,不必言告于我,只要将你带来的谷子倒入粮仓,就可以取走相同容量的杏子。"董奉用杏子换取来的谷子救济庐山周围的贫苦老百姓和接济旅途上断绝了盘缠的路人,每年多达两万余人。

看到这些神奇的事,人们就更加感谢董奉了,从此,"杏林"一词,也就流传衍变为中医药的代名词了。

When the apricots were ripe, Dong Feng built a barn in the woods. People were told, "those who want to buy apricots just put the same amount of millet into the barn as that of the apricots and take them away." Dong Feng exchanged apricots for millet to relieve the poor around Lushan Mountain and also passers-by who had no more money for their journey. Every year, more than 20,000 people were helped in this manner.

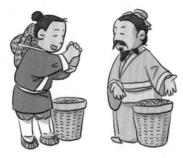

Seeing such magnanimity, people were even more grateful to Dong Feng. Since then, the word "Apricot wood" has become a synonym for TCM.

第十二章　悬壶济世的传说

　　东汉时有个叫费长房的人。非常渴望学习医术,可是苦于没有老师教授,一天,他在酒楼喝酒解闷,看见街上有一位卖药的老翁,悬挂着一个药葫芦兜售丸散膏丹,效果很好,来买药的人络绎不绝。而且,老翁乐善好施,对待看不起病的穷苦人就免费送药,大家都交口称赞。

　　费长房看了好几天,断定这位老翁医术精湛,绝非等闲之辈。他买了酒肉,恭恭敬敬地拜见老翁,表达了想学习医术的来意,老翁看他十分诚心,便让他随自己学习,经过多年的学习,费长房终于学成了,临行之际,老翁特地将药葫芦赠送给他,要他用医术救济百姓。

Chapter 12 The Legend of Hanging a Gourd to Cure the Sick

There was a man named Fei Zhangfang in the Eastern Han dynasty, who was eager to learn medicine, but had no one to teach him. One day, when he was drinking alcohol in a restaurant to relieve his boredom, he saw an old man selling medicine on the street, hanging on his walking stick a medicine gourd with pills, powders and pellets, which proved effective to patients. Therefore, people came to buy his medicine one after another. What's more, the old man was generous and gave free medicine to the poor who could not afford the medical fees, which was praised by everyone.

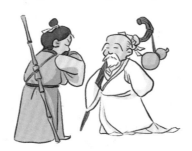

Fei Zhangfang watched the old man for several days and decided that he had superb medical skills and was by no means an ordinary person. He bought some alcohol and meat, respectfully visited the old man, and expressed his desire to learn medicine. Seeing his sincerity, the old man allowed him to learn from himself. After years of study, Fei Zhangfang finally became a doctor. Before leaving, the old man specially presented him with a medicine gourd, asking Fei to use his medicine to help people suffering from illnesses.

费长房回到家后,便开始行医治病,治病时手到病除,没有不好的。为了纪念老师,他便在腰间悬挂一个葫芦,这便是悬葫济世的由来。

后来,民间的郎中为了纪念这个传奇式的医师,就在药铺门口挂一个药葫芦作为行医的标志。如今,虽然中医大夫"悬壶"已很少见到,但"悬壶"这一说法保留了下来。

After Fei Zhangfang returned home, he began to practice medicine. As an excellent doctor, he could always cure his patients immediately, with no exception. In memory of his teacher, he hung a gourd on his waist, hence the origin of "hanging a gourd to help the sick".

Later, in memory of this legendary doctor, a medicine gourd is hung at the door of pharmacy as a sign of practicing medicine. Nowadays, although the "hanging a gourd" of doctors of TCM is rarely seen, the saying has been kept on.

第十三章　张仲景与"饺子"

东汉末年,各地灾害严重,很多人身患疾病。名医张仲景不仅医术高明,而且医德高尚,无论穷人和富人他都认真治疗,救了无数的性命。

张仲景在长沙当官时,就经常在大堂上为百姓看病,这就是"坐堂大夫"的由来,有一年冬天到了,他看到很多穷苦百姓忍饥受寒,耳朵都冻烂了,心里非常难受,想要帮助他们。他叫弟子在空地上搭起棚子,架起大锅,在冬至那天,向穷人发放药物治冻伤。张仲景的药名叫"祛(qū)寒娇耳汤",做法是用羊肉、生姜、大葱和一些祛寒药材在锅里煮熬,煮好后再把这些东西捞出来切碎,用面皮包成耳朵状的"娇耳",下锅煮熟后分给求药的病人。每人两只娇耳,一碗汤。人们吃下祛寒汤后浑身发热,两只耳朵变得暖和起来。吃了一段时间,病人冻烂的耳朵就好了。

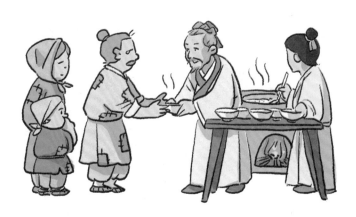

Chapter 13 Zhang Zhongjing and "Dumplings"

At the end of the Eastern Han dynasty, severe disasters were common everywhere and many people suffered from diseases. Zhang Zhongjing, a famous doctor, not only had excellent medical skills, but also noble medical ethics. He treated both the poor and the rich seriously and saved countless lives.

When serving as an official in Changsha, Zhang Zhongjing often treated the common people in his hall, which gave rise to the term "hall (clinic) doctor". One winter, he saw many poor people suffering from hunger and cold, with their ears frozen. He felt very sad and wanted to help them. He told his students to build a shed in an open space, set up a cauldron, and on the day of the winter solstice, distributed medicine to the poor to treat their frostbites. The name of Zhang Zhongjing's medicine is *Quhan Jiao'er Decoction* (clod-dispelling and ear-remedying soup), which was made by boiling mutton, ginger, green onions and some cold-dispelling medicinal materials in a pot. After being boiled, these ingredients were fished out and chopped, wrapped into ear-shaped "Jiao'er" with dough, later cooked in the pot and distributed to patients seeking medicine. Each person was given two "ears" and a bowl of soup. After eating the cold dispelling soup with the "ears", people felt hot all over and their ears became warm. Eating that soup for a period of time, their frozen ears were finally cured.

061

　　张仲景发药一直持续到大年三十，大年初一，人们庆祝新年，也庆祝烂耳朵变好，就模仿"娇耳"的样子做过年的食物，并在初一早上吃。人们称这种食物为"饺耳""饺子"或"扁食"，在冬至和大年初一吃，以纪念张仲景开棚发药和治病的日子。慢慢的，冬至吃饺子防冻耳朵的风俗便流传了下来。

　　今天，虽然我们用不着用"娇耳"来治冻烂的耳朵了，但饺子却已成了人们最常见、最爱吃的食品。

Zhang Zhongjing kept distributing medicine until the Chinese New Year's Eve. On the Chinese New Year's Day, people celebrated the New Year and the healing of their frozen ears. They made food by modeling after the appearance of "Jiao Er", and served themselves with it on the morning of the New Year's Day. People called this kind of food "dumpling ear", "dumpling" or "flat food", which is the main thing to eat on the winter solstice and the Lunar New Year's Day, to commemorate the day when Zhang Zhongjing opened the shed to distribute medicine and cure diseases. Slowly, the custom of eating dumplings to prevent frozen ears on the winter solstice came down.

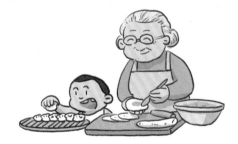

Nowadays, though we do not need to eat "Jiao Er" to cure frozen ears, dumplings have become a most common and favorite food for people.

第十四章　药王孙思邈

孙思邈,陕西耀县人,是中国历史上不多的年过百岁的老人之一。

孙思邈小时候体弱多病,家中为他看病而花光了积蓄,于是他从小就下定决心,要成为一名医生,为天下的穷人看病救命。经过多年的刻苦学习,孙思邈医术达到了很高的水平。他谢绝了皇帝让他当太医的邀请,而是继续在百姓中间,治病救人,著书立说。

Chapter 14 Sun Simiao, China's King of Medicine

Sun Simiao, a native of Yaoxian County, Shaanxi Province, was one of the few centenarians in Chinese history.

As a child, Sun Simiao was weak and sick, and his family spent all their savings on the medical treatment for him. Therefore, he made up his mind from an early age to become a doctor and save the lives of the poor. After years of hard study, Sun gained superb medical skills. He declined the emperor's invitation to be an imperial physician and stayed among the common people to cure them and save their lives. He also wrote some medical books claiming his opinions.

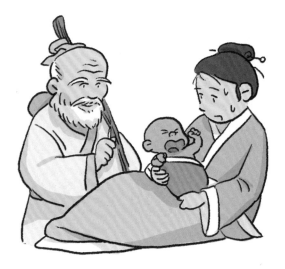

有一次,孙思邈在路上看到四个人抬着一口棺材往前走,殷红的鲜血从棺材缝里滴下地来,后面跟了一个老婆婆,哭得死去活来。孙思邈上前探问,原来是老婆婆的女儿因难产折腾了两天两夜,孩子没有生下来,女儿的命却丢掉了。孙思邈问明了这女子才死了没有几个时辰,于是要求老婆婆把棺材打开,他试着救救看。棺材打开后,孙思邈仔细摸了摸脉,感觉到还有一丝跳动。于是赶紧选好穴位,针刺起来,不一会儿,妇人的胸部有了起伏,腹部也蠕动起来。"哇!——"随着一声婴儿的啼哭声,一个白白胖胖的娃娃生了下来,产妇也睁开了双眼。孙思邈赶紧把随身带的药拿了出来,给产妇喂了下去。不一会儿产妇便完全苏醒过来。孙思邈一根针救活了母子俩的性命,人们都称赞他是神医。

One day, Sun Simiao saw on a road four people carrying a coffin, with red blood dripping from the cracks of the coffin, which was followed by an old woman, crying her eyes out. Sun stepped forward to inquire on what had happened. It turned out that the old woman's daughter had been tossing about for two days and two nights due to a difficult childbirth. Ultimately, the baby was not born, and her daughter died. Learning that the woman had only been "dead" for a few hours, Sun asked to have the coffin opened, and examined to see if he could save her. After the coffin was opened, Sun felt her pulse carefully and found that there was still a trace of beating. Finding the exact acupuncture point at once, he inserted the needle into it. Before long, the woman began to breathe again, and there was a wriggle in her abdomen. With a loud cry, a plump baby was born, and the mother opened her eyes. Sun Simiao quickly took out the medicine he had along with him and fed it to the new mother. After a while, she came to life completely. The news that Sun Simiao saved the life of a mother and a baby with a needle immediately spread around, and people praised him as a miracle doctor.

有一天,孙思邈替一个腿痛的人治病。他开了汤药,病人服后无效。他又配合做针刺疗法,扎了几次,病人还是喊痛。他想,除了书上讲的穴位外,难道没有别的新穴位？于是他一面用大拇指在病人腿上轻轻地掐,一面问病人:"是不是这儿痛?"掐着掐着,病人忽然叫了起来:"啊!是,是这儿!"孙思邈就在这个部位扎了一针,病人的腿痛果然止住了。

孙思邈想,书上没有这个穴位,取个什么名呢？噢,对了,病人说"啊!是……"那就叫"阿是"穴好了。孙思邈所创用的以痛取位的"阿是"穴,是他对发展针灸学的一大贡献,已被千余年来无数针灸学者所验证肯定。

One day, when treating a man with pains in his leg, Sun Simiao prescribed a decoction, but it had no effect. He gave acupuncture therapy and pricked several times, but the patient still cried out for pain. He thought, "Besides the acupoints mentioned in the book, aren't there other undiscovered acupoints?" So he pinched the patient's leg gently with his thumb and asked the patient, "Does it hurt here?"Upon his pinching, the patient suddenly cried out,"Ouch, Yes, that's it!" Sun Simiao pricked a needle into this part, and the pain in the patient's leg indeed stopped.

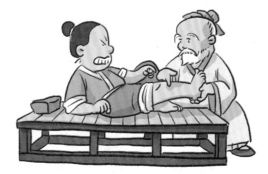

Sun Simiao thought,"there is no such acupoint recorded in the book, what shall I name it?" "Ouch, Yes!", that's what the patient said. So let me call it "Ashi Point" (similar in pronuciation to "ouch"). The "Ashi" acupoint discovered and named by Sun, fixing the point according to the pain, is a great contribution to the development of acupuncture, and it has been verified and affirmed by numerous acupuncture scholars for more than a thousand years.

孙思邈70岁时编写了《千金要方》一书，收医方四千多首，又过了三十年，百岁老人孙思邈深感《千金要方》不足以全面反映自己的心得体会和新获得的珍贵医药学知识，续撰《千金翼方》，收医方两千多首。"翼"就是辅助的意思，用以补充前一部书的不足。

孙思邈被后人尊称为"药王"，他故乡附近有座他经常采药的山被称为药王山，山上还建有药王庙。

At the age of 70 years old, Sun Simiao compiled the *Qianjin Yao Fang* (*Essential Prescriptions for Emergencies*), collecting in it more than 4,000 medical prescriptions. Thirty years later, Sun Simiao, a centenarian, deeply felt that the book was not adequate to fully reflect his own experience and newly acquired precious medical knowledge. He continued to write the *Qianjin Yi Fang* (*Essential Prescriptions*), which collected more than 2,000 medical prescriptions. "Yi (Wing)" means supplement, which was meant to remedy the shortcomings of his previous book.

Sun Simiao was honored as the "China's king of medicine (an excellent herblist)" by later generations. Near his hometown, the mountain where he often went to collect herbs was named the Mountain of the China's king of medicine. A Temple with the same name was also built on the mountain.

第十五章　吴师机与狗皮膏药

　　膏药疗法是中医传统的外治疗法,清代吴师机是一位擅长膏药疗法且卓有成就的医生。

　　吴师机开始行医后发现膏药疗法具有简单、便捷、廉价、效果明显的优点,又可避免内服药所引起的副作用,特别是穷苦人家用膏药效果很好还很便宜,于是他在百姓中大力推行膏药。由于膏药疗法不分老幼,仅一张膏药贴敷就能取得很好的效果,而且不影响劳作,所以深得广大劳苦百姓喜欢,应诊者络绎不绝。

　　吴师机不仅医技精湛,而且医德高尚,为人乐善好施。当时到他家看病的人每天都有五六十船,最多的时候一个月曾治两万多人次。他还在扬州开设药局,专门以自制膏药赠送病家,广受当地群众赞誉。

Chapter 15 Wu Shiji and Therapy Plaster

Plaster therapy has been a covential external treatment in Traditional Chinese Medicine (TCM). In the Qing dynasty, there was a successful doctor named Wu Shiji, who was good at plaster therapy.

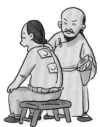

After he began to practice medicine, Wu Shiji found that plaster therapy had the advantages of being simple, convenient, cheap and effective, and could avoid the side effects caused by oral administration, especially suitable for poor people who could afford it! So he vigorously promoted this therapy among the people. Because plaster therapy could be used for treating both men and women of all ages. Just one plaster can achieve desirable effect without suspending regular labor, so it was deeply loved by the working people, and sought by an endless stream of patients.

Wu Shiji had excellent medical skills, as well as noble medical ethics and a kind heart. In those days, fifty or so boatloads of patients came to his home every day. A maximum of more than 20,000 patients were treated in a month. He also set up pharmacies in Yangzhou for the common people, presenting self-made plasters to them, his deeds thus being widely praised by the local people.

　　吴师机对医学的一大贡献在于他将自己的外治经验著成《理瀹(yuè)骈(pián)文》,书中介绍了外治法的历史,阐述了外治法的理论根据,以及膏药的制法、用法和治疗范围、作用。该书最大的特色是打破了以往医生偏于药饵轻于外治的惯例,大力推崇外治疗法,其中突出膏药疗法。

　　该书一问世,就因实用性和可靠性,深受同行好评,当时上海、山东、安徽等地的医生都纷纷效仿他的医技,不少药铺还专门编印他书中的医方和制药方法。吴师机对发展中医的外治法作出了杰出贡献,故后人尊称他为外治之宗。

One of Wu's great contributions to medicine is his work *Li Yue Pianwen* (*A Rhymed Discourse on External Remedies*), in which he introduced the history of external treatment, elaborated on its theoretical basis, as well as the preparation, usage, scope and function of plasters. The main feature of his book is that he broke the convention that doctors preferred oral administration to external treatment, and strongly advocated external treatment, in which the plaster therapy was highlighted.

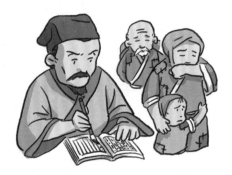

Soon after its publication, the book was highly praised by his peers for its practicality and reliability. And doctors in Shanghai, Shandong, Anhui and other places imitated his medical skills one after another, and many pharmacies specially compiled and printed out the medical prescriptions and pharmaceutical methods from his book. Wu Shiji has made outstanding contributions to the development of external treatment in TCM, so later generations have respectfully called him the "Master of External Treatment".

第四单元　古今中医药学教育

由于中医药学学科的特殊性,中医从业者需要持续的教育和学习,在几千年的发展过程中,中医药学的教育模式不断演化改变,从古至今,名医辈出。

远古时期,我们的祖先在长期生活和生产中发现了医药知识,并开始以口传心授的形式传播中医药知识。随着医药知识经验的增多,口传心授被家族和师徒相传的中医教育形式取代,久而久之就形成了很多中医流派和中医世家,同时也造就了很多名医。

Unit Ⅳ Traditional Chinese Medicine Education in Ancient and Modern Times

A practitioner of Traditional Chinese Medicine (TCM) needs continuous education and learning due to its the specialty of TCM. In the course of thousands of years, the education mode of TCM has been constantly evolving and changing. From ancient times to the present, famous doctors have emerged in large numbers.

In ancient times, the Chinese ancestors acquried medical knowledge in their long-term of living and production, and began to spread the knowledge of TCM in the form of oral instruction. With the increase in medical knowledge and experience, oral instruction has been replaced by TCM education handed down from family members on or from a master to his apprentices. Over time, many schools and families of TCM have come into being, and many famous doctors thus appeared.

077

随着社会的发展和人类健康要求的不断提高，官办的中医教育机构相继出现，从唐代开始，历朝历代都设有专门的中央和地方官办医学教育机构，辛亥革命后，开始举办具有现代教育模式的中医学校，民国期间全国各地先后建立了多间规模较大的中医学校。

中华人民共和国成立后，中国的中医药事业迎来了生机勃发的春天，从20世纪50年代开始，全国各地创建了一批中医药大学，中医课程进入了医学高等教育中，从此开始了中医药专业人员现代教育模式的新历程。

With the development of the society and increasing needs for better health, officially-run TCM education institutions emerged one after another. Since the Tang dynasty, there had been special central and local government-run medical education institutions in all periods. After the Revolution of 1911, schools with modern education models began to be set up. During the period of the Republic of China (1912-1949), many large-scale schools were established across the country.

After the founding of the People's Republic of China, TCM in China ushered in a vigorous spring. Since the 1950s, a number of TCM universities have been established, and relevant courses entered into the higher medical education system. Thereupon, a modern education mode for TCM professionals has been carried on.

第十六章　古代中医的教育

中医药学已经在中国发展了几千年，它的教育方式，大约有家传、师带徒、学堂、学校以及大学五种模式。

远古时期，我们的祖先在长期生活和生产中发现了医药知识，相应地产生了最原始的医学教育形式：口传心授。随着社会分工的出现和医药知识经验的增多，口传心授被家族和师徒相传的中医教育形式取代。由于世代相传的医疗经验的积累，知识更加专业化，久而久之就形成了很多中医专科和中医世家，同时也造就了很多名医。比如：古代著名医家徐之才，他们家族世代行医，六代之中就有十一个名医。家传式的中医教育形式一直被后世沿用下来。

Chapter 16 Traditional Chinese Medicine Education in Ancient China

Traditional Chinese Medicine (TCM) has developed for thousands of years in China, and there have been five modes of education in it: family education, apprenticeship education, private school education, public school education and university education.

In ancient times, medical knowledge was acquired and accumulated by our ancestors in their lives and production. Accordingly, the most primitive mode of medical education was via verbal and mental instruction. With the emergence of social division of labor and the increase in medical knowledge and experience, verbal and mental instruction was replaced by the mode of family and apprenticeship education. With the accumulation of medical experience handed down from generation to generation in one family, knowledge was more specialized. Over time, many TCM specialties and families practising medicine for generations emerged, so did many famous doctors. For example, Xu Zhicai, a famous doctor in the Qi of the Northern dynasties (550-557) whose family practiced TCM for six generations with eleven famous doctors emerging. And the mode of family education has continued till the present.

伴随家传式中医教育出现的是名医带徒教育,这种中医教育形式扩大了医学流传的范围,有利于培养更多的医家,适应了民众防治疾病的需求。许多医家在传授时结合自己的经验,以自己的见解发挥前人的学术,相继各树一帜,各成一说,从而形成了不同的中医流派,促进了医学的争论、交流与发展。

古代名医在接收徒弟时都要经过十分精心的挑选,要求徒弟聪慧、勤奋、诚信,并且有良好的品德,而弟子为了寻求名师,更是不辞辛劳,遍地求访。

Family education in TCM was accompanied by the emergence of apprenticeship education, which had expanded the scope of medical communication, promoted the doctor's training, and met more public needs for disease prevention and treatment. Many doctors combined their experience with their own interpretations of the academic achievements of their predecessors in their instruction. Thus, there emerged different schools of TCM, promoting the debates on, communication and development of medicine.

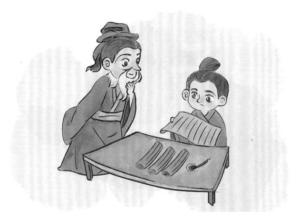

Famous doctors in ancient times would carefully select their students, accroding to the following criteria: intelligence, diligence, honesty and virtue. And a practitioner-to-be would spare no effort to go anywhere in order to seek for a famous doctor to be his teacher.

随着历史发展,政府办的中医教育机构就出现了。在唐代,当时有中央与地方两级医学教育制度。中央级称为"太医署",规模很大,有师生三、四百人;地方上均开办医学,各地普遍设置医学博士和医学助教。宋代设"太医局",有学生三百余人,学习内容分九个科,这时的教育方针重视实习训练,强调从临床中获取知识经验。

元明清时期的医学教育大体上也是继承宋以来的体制,由太医院管理医学教育。鸦片战争后,官办的中医教育已徒具形式,在中医人才培养上已基本不起作用了。

辛亥革命后,中国中医界开始举办具有现代教育模式的中医学校,全国各地先后建立了多间规模较大的中医学校,形成了近现代中医教育的高潮。

With the development of history, institutions for TCM education run by the government emerged. In the Tang dynasty, there was a two-tier medical education system, i.e. in the central and local government. At the central level, the institution was called the "Imperial Medical Department", which was of a very large scale, with 300 or 400 teachers and students. At the local level, medical education institutions were everywhere with numerous medical doctors and assistants. In the Song dynasty, the "Imperial Medical Bureau" was set up, with more than 300 students, and the learning content was divided into nine subjects. At that time, the medical education attached importance to practical training, emphasizing the acquisition of knowledge and experience from clinical practices.

Medical education in the Yuan, Ming and Qing dynasties generally inherited the system from the Song dynasty. Imperial Hospital was in charge of medical education. After the First Opium War, the official education institutions had become a mere formality, and they had basically no effect on the training of Chinese medical talents.

After the Revolution of 1911, TCM communities began to set up schools with modern education modes. Many large-scale schools have been established throughout the country, giving rise to a climax of modern Chinese medicine education.

第十七章 王惟一和针灸铜人的故事

随着中医在世界上的传播,针灸和推拿慢慢也走出国门,拔罐的痕迹也是常常出现在外国人的肩膀上、胳膊上。而这一切都离不开中医教育传承,其中,对针灸教育贡献最大的医家便是王惟一。

王惟一生活在宋代,那个时候由于针灸学由于没有统一的规范,导致一些穴位的定位标记错误了,这样学生也学错了。于是王惟一便著成医书《铜人腧穴针灸图经》,规范了针灸图谱,订正错误。还将全书内容刻在石头上,以便人们学习。这是世界上首次由政府颁布的针灸标准。

Chapter 17 The Story of Wang Weiyi and the Acupuncture and Bronze Figure

With the spread of Traditional Chinese Medicine (TCM) to the world, acupuncture and moxibustion have gradually gone out. Traces of cupping therapy are often seen on the shoulders and arms of foreigners, too. All of these cannot be separated from the inheritance of TCM education. It's well acknowledged that Wang Weiyi was the doctor who has made the greatest contribution to acupuncture education.

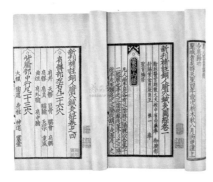

《铜人腧穴针灸图经》古籍
An Ancient Version of the *Tongren Shuxue Zhenjiu Tu Jing* (*Illustrated Manual of Acu - puncture Points on the Bronze Figure*)

Wang Weiyi lived in the Song dynasty, when, because there was no uniform standard for acupuncture and moxibustion, the positioning marks of some acupoints were wrong, and hence the students also learned the wrong ways. Therefore, Wang wrote the *Tongren Shuxue Zhenjiu Tu Jing* (*Illustrated Manual of Acupuncture Points on the Bronze Figure*), which standardized the atlas of acupuncture points and corrected previous errors. And he carved the contents of the book on stones so that people could learn them. This is the first government-issued acupuncture standards in the world.

　　王惟一的另一巨大贡献是铸成了人体针灸铜人,针灸铜人均仿成年男子而制,躯壳由前后两件构成,内置脏腑,外刻腧穴,各穴均与体内相通,外涂黄蜡,内灌水或水银,刺中穴位,则液体溢出,稍差则针不能入,因而可使医生按此试针,以供教学和考试之用。针灸铜人与《铜人腧穴针灸图经》相辅行世,让当时学习医术的人有了清晰的可以参考的资料,让针灸事业得到了发展,对针灸学的发展起到了极大的贡献。

Another great contribution of Wang Weiyi was to cast a Bronze Figure for practicing acupuncture, in imitation of an adult male body, which was composed of two parts, one in front and the other in back. The viscera were built inside, and the acupoints were carved on the outside, with each acupoint being connected with the body. Yellow wax was coated on the outside, and water or mercury was filled in. If the acupoint was punctured in the right manner, liquid would flow out of it, and if wrongly punctured, the needle could not pierce in. Therefore, doctors can use the above model for needle trial, which can be used for teaching and examination.The *Acupuncture Bronze Figure* and the *Tongren Shuxue Zhenjiu Tu Jing* together propelled progress in acupuncture and moxibustion, thus making marvellous contributions to their development.

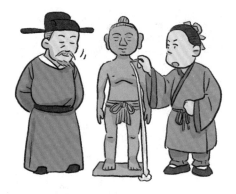

第十八章 李时珍与《本草纲目》

李时珍是明代伟大的医药学家、博物学家。出生于医学世家,李时珍自幼攻读四书五经,十三岁时考取秀才。矢志以医药为业。李时珍因医术高明,在乡里颇负盛名,曾治愈蕲州富顺王、武昌楚王之子,医名大振。二十七岁时,其被推荐赴京城太医院任职,他借此阅读了大量珍贵的医书,发现既往中药书中有很多错误,他忧心忡忡,毅然辞职归乡,决心重新编写一部内容翔实的中药学著作。

李时珍在家里闭门读书十多年,阅读了大量有关中药学、植物学、医学、农学等著作,他为了准确描述药物的形状,深入山林、田野、矿井,实地考察,足迹遍及河北、河南、江西、安徽、江苏等地,虚心求教,亲自采集药物,认真比对,历经三十年时间,编成了药物学巨著《本草纲目》。

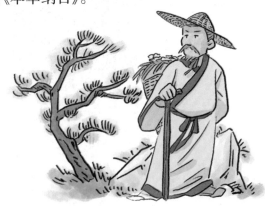

Chapter 18 Li Shizhen and *A Compendium of Materia Medica*

Li Shizhen was a great medical scientist and naturalist in the Ming dynasty. Born in a family that had practiced medicine for generations, Li studied the *Four Books* and *Five Classics* (The Confucius Classics) at an early age and passed the imperial examination at the county level at the age of 13. He determined to devote himself to the research on medical science. Li became famous in his village because of his excellent medical skills. He once cured King Fushun of Qizhou and the son of King Chu of Wuchang, thus gaining a great fame as a doctor. At the age of 27, he was recommended to work in the Imperial Hospital of capital. He read a large number of precious medical books there and found that there were many errors in previous books on materia medica, so he resigned and returned home, and decided to compile a new book with detailed contents.

After returning home, Li Shizhen devoted himself to reading for more than 10 years, reading a lot of books on Traditional Chinese Medicine (TCM), botany, medicine, agronomy, etc. He went deep into mountain forests, fields and mines and traveled to Hebei, Henan, Jiangxi, Anhui, Jiangsu and other provinces. He made on-the-spot investigations, sought advice modestly, collected herbs in person, and carefully identified them. Working hard for 30 years, he finally finished the great work the *Bencao Gangmu* (*A Compendium of Materia Medica*).

　　《本草纲目》共收药物1892种,其中李时珍新增药物374种,还附有1109幅精美插图。是中国历史上记载药物最多,插图最多的一部本草著作。全书共190多万字,分为各种类别共60类。李时珍对每种药物进行了详细地注解,既保存了历代本草文献,也记述了丰富的实践经验。《本草纲目》从实用出发,在药物后面还附有相应的方剂。全书共收集各种方剂达11 096首,其中多数是李时珍自身实践和收集所得。

　　《本草纲目》是一本有世界性影响的著作,很早就传到日本、朝鲜、越南等国,并被翻译成多种文字介绍到世界各地。生物学家达尔文称赞《本草纲目》是"中国古代的百科全书"。著名科学史家李约瑟在《中国科学技术史》中高度评价这本书:"毫无疑问,明代最伟大的科学成就,就是李时珍那部登峰造极的《本草纲目》。"

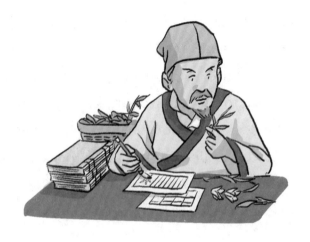

The *Bencao Gangmu* lists 1892 species of materia medicas of 60 categories, of which 374 were added in by Li Shizhen. With more than 1.9 million characters in it, the *Bencao Gangmu*, was the most illustrated book and recorded the largest number of herbs in Chinese history. Li Shizhen annotated each medicine in detail, which not only preserved the herbal literature of past dynasties, but also recorded rich practical experience. The *Bencao Gangmu* aims at practical use, and contains prescriptions after descriptions of herbs. There are 11, 096 prescriptions in the whole book, most of which came from Li Shizhen's own practice and collection.

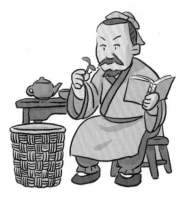

The *Bencao Gangmu*, a work of worldwide influence, was introduced to Japan, Korea, Vietnam and other countries very early and have been translated into many languages and introduced to all other parts of the world. Darwin, a biologist, praised the *Bencao Gangmu* as "an encyclopedia of ancient China". Joseph Needham, a famous sinologist, spoke highly of Li Shizhen's *Bencao Gangmu* in his *History of Science and Civilization in China*,"There is no doubt that the greatest scientific achievement of the Ming dynasty is Li Shizhen's *Bencao Gangmu*."

第十九章　现代中医药教育

中华人民共和国成立以来,中医药高等教育从无到有、从弱到强,经过一代代中医药人的不懈努力,中医药高等教育实现了跨越式发展。

自 1956 年国务院批准设立北京、上海、广州、成都四所中医学院以来,中医药高等教育已经走过了 60 多年的历程,目前全国有高等中医药院校 42 所,其中独立设置的本科中医药高等院校 25 所,院校教育已成为中医药高等教育的主体,实现了由传统教育方式向现代教育方式的转变,初步形成了以院校教育为主体,多层次、多类型协调发展的办学格局。

Chapter 19 Modern Chinese Medicine Education

Since the founding of the People's Republic of China, the higher education of Traditional Chinese Medicine (TCM) has grown out of almost nothing. Through the unremitting efforts of several generations of TCM practitioners, leapfrog achievements have been made in it.

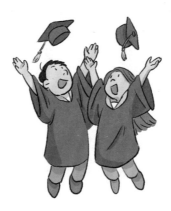

Since the establishment of four colleges of TCM in Beijing, Shanghai, Guangzhou and Chengdu approved by State Council in 1956, the higher education of TCM has undergone a development of more than 60 years. At present, there are 42 colleges and universities of TCM in China, of which 25 are independent undergraduate colleges or universities. College education has become the main body of higher education in TCM. It has realized a transformation from traditional education modes to modern education ones, and basically formed a multi-level and multi-type coordinated pattern featuring college education as the main part.

近年来,中医药大学通过院校教育与师承教育相结合的中医药人才培养模式,培养了一大批中医药传承创新人才。

目前,中医药类专业在校生数已达到70余万人,为中医药医疗、保健、科研、教育、产业、文化及对外交流与合作等各个领域提供了高质量的专业人才,为构建我国独具特色的医药卫生体系和推动中医药事业发展作出了重要贡献。

为传承民族医药文化、培养民族医药人才,全国开办了不同形式的民族医药相关教育培训。仅2011—2015年期间就培养了5000余名民族医药专业人才,促进了民族医药传承与发展。

In recent years, universities of TCM have carried out reform in talent training modes through a combination of traditional master-student teaching with college education, cultivating a large number of innovative figures of TCM.

At present, the number of students majoring in TCM has reached more than 700,000, providing high-quality professionals for various fields such as medical treatment, health care, scientific research, education, industry, cultural and external exchange and cooperation. They make great contributions to the construction of China's unique medical and health system and the promotion of further development of TCM.

In order to inherit the culture of ethnic medicine and train talents in those aspects, different forms of education and programs related to ethnic medicines have been launched throughout the country. During the "12th Five-Year Plan" period (2011-2015) alone, more than 5000 ethnic medicine professionals were produced, helping promote the inheritance and development of the medicine of different ethnic groups.

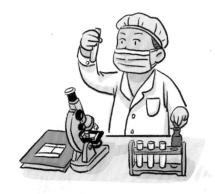

第二十章 留学生与中医药

近年来,随着中国教育对外开放的不断加深以及世界各国对中医药的认可度不断提高,中医药已传播到183个国家和地区。中医药院校在各大洲建立了中医孔子学院、海外中医中心等对外交流合作机构,开展了不同形式的教育合作项目,为推进中医药国际化进程、传播中华优秀传统文化、提升国家软实力作出了积极贡献。

多年来,来华学习中医药的留学生一直居来华学习自然科学留学人数的首位。经教育部批准,全国有20多所高等中医药院校具备接受外国留学生的资格。外国留学生、进修生学成归国,用所学的中医药知识为本国人民健康服务,扩大了中医药在国际上的影响,推动了中医药的国际交流与合作。

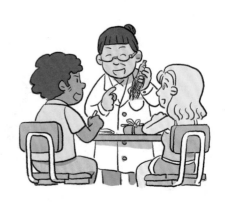

Chapter 20 Overseas Students and Traditional Chinese Medicine

In recent years, with the deepening opening up of China's education and the increasing recognition in the world. Traditional Chinese Medicine (TCM) has spread to 183 countries and regions. Colleges and universities of TCM have established Confucius Institutes of TCM, overseas Chinese medicine centers and other exchange and cooperation facilities on different continents, which have carried out various forms of educational cooperation projects, thus making positive contributions to promoting the internationalization of TCM, disseminating excellent traditional Chinese culture and, in a way, enhancing the soft power of China.

Over the years, the number of foreign students studying TCM in China has always ranked the greatest among those coming to China for studying natural sciences. With the approval of the Ministry of Education of China, more than 20 Chinese colleges and universities of TCM are now qualified to accept foreign students. Those who finished their study in China have returned to their motherlands and are now in service of people's health in their own countries with their knowledge of TCM, thus expanding the influence of TCM around the world and promoting international exchange and cooperation in medicine.

目前,130个国家的中医医疗机构有5万多家,针灸师超过10万人,注册中医师超过2万人。在中医学术活动方面,国外有许多国际性和地域性的中医药学术组织,创办了中医药杂志并经常承办学术活动。中医在泰国、新加坡等国已得到立法保护,中药已在多个国家获得批准对治疗药品进行注册。全球接受过中医药、针灸、推拿等治疗的人数已到世界总人口的三分之一以上。

世界中医药教育在近几十年来得到很大的发展,不少西方国家的大学已经开始举办中医药教育,中医药教育的国际化局面正在形成,日本、韩国、英国、德国、法国、澳大利亚、美国等国都建立了政府承认的中医药高等医学院校。

Up until now, there have been more than 50,000 TCM institutions in more than 130 countries, with more than 100,000 acupuncturists and more than 20,000 registered TCM doctors. In terms of academic activities, there are many international and regional TCM organizations around the world, which have launched journals on TCM and carried out regular academic activities. TCM has been protected by legislation in countries like Thailand and Singapore. Registration of TCM pharmaceuticals have been approved in some countries. The number of people who turn to TCM, acupuncture, massage and other treatments has accounted for more than one third of the world's population.

Education in TCM has developed greatly in recent decades around the world. Many official universities in western countries have begun to teach TCM, and the internationalization of TCM education is taking shape. Medical colleges and universities have been approved and set up by governments in Japan, Korea, Britain, Germany, France, Australia and the United States.

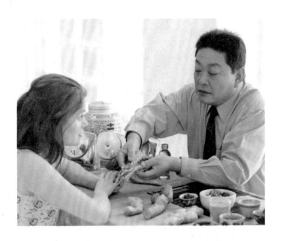

第五单元　中医药学对世界的贡献

中医药学发展了几千年,很多治疗技术随着文化交流扩散到世界各地,为世界各国的医学发展作出了一定的贡献。

早在秦汉时期,中医药就传到朝鲜、日本、越南。到了唐代,不少国家派人来中国学习中医药。宋代与海外50多个国家通商,外运的中药品种、数量都大量增加。《马可波罗游记》记载了大量中药被商人运往亚丁,再转运到北非的亚历山大等地。

Unit V The Contribution of Traditional Chinese Medicine to the World

Traditional Chinese medicine (TCM) has developed for thousands of years, and many of its treatment techniques have spread to all parts of the world with cultural exchanges, making more or less contributions to the medical development of all countries in the world.

As early as the Qin and Han dynasties, TCM was spread to Korea, Japan, and Vietnam. In the Tang dynasty, many countries sent people to China to study TCM. In the Song dynasty, more than 50 overseas countries developed trade with China with greater varieties and quantities of Chinese medicines exported. *The Travels of Marco Polo* records that a large number of Chinese medicines were transported by merchants to Aden, and then to Alexandria and other places in North Africa.

中国的医家们很早就注意天花的治疗研究，而且积极采取预防措施。到了明代，随着对传染性疾病的认识加深和治疗痘疹的经验越来越丰富，医家们发明了人痘接种术，这是对人类健康的重大贡献。中药走向全世界最突出的成果是中国的青蒿素惠及全球，每年挽救上万人的生命，被誉为"20世纪后半叶最伟大的医学创举"。

随着社会发展，慢性疾病不断增多，人们的健康观念发生了变化。在世界范围内，回归自然、重视传统医药已经成为重要的趋势，传统医药在全球日益受到更多的关注。

Chinese doctors have been dedicated to the research on the treatment of smallpox much earlier and took active preventive measures against it. In the Ming dynasty, with the deeper understanding of infectious diseases and richer experience in the treatment of pox, variolation was invented, having helped improve human health. The most outstanding outcome brought about by Chinese herbal medicines going to the world is artemisinin, which has benefited the world and saved thousands of lives, and is called the greatest pioneering medical achievement in the second half of 20th century.

With the development of society and the rise of chronic diseases, people's health concepts have also been changed. It has become an important trend to return to nature and attach more importance to traditional medicine in the world.

第二十一章　屠呦呦与青蒿素的故事

2015 年，中国女科学家屠呦（yōu）呦因为发现了青蒿素成为第一位获得诺贝尔奖的中国科学家。

屠呦呦出生于浙江省宁波市。名字来源于中国最早的诗歌总集——《诗经》里"呦呦鹿鸣，食野之苹"的名句，寄托了父母对她的美好期待。1951 年，屠呦呦考入北京大学药学系，毕业后从事中药研究，取得了许多骄人的成果。其中，研制用于治疗疟疾的药物——青蒿素，是她最杰出的成就。

疟疾是一种严重危害人类生命健康的世界性流行病。世界卫生组织报告，全世界约数 10 亿人口生活在疟疾流行区，每年约 2 亿人患疟疾，数百余万人被夺去生命。中国从 1964 年重新开始对抗疟新药进行研究，从中草药中寻求突破是整个工作的主流，但是，通过对数千种中草药的筛选，却没有任何重要发现。

Chapter 21 The Story of Tu Youyou and Artemisinin

In 2015, Tu Youyou became the first native Chinese scientist to win a Nobel Prize for her discovery of artemisinin.

Tu Youyou was born in Ningbo, Zhejiang Province. Her name comes from the famous line in the *Book of Songs* (a collection of ancient poems), the earliest collection of poems in China, "Yoyo, a herd of deer are bellowing and gazing wild Artemisia". Her name expresses her parents' best wishes for her. In 1951, Tu was admitted to the Department of Pharmacy in Peking University. After graduation, she has been engaged in the research on Chinese herbal medicines and made multiple remarkable achievements, of which the discovery of artemisinin, a drug used to fight against malaria, is the most outstanding one.

Malaria has been a worldwide epidemic that seriously endangers human health and life. The WHO reports that about one billion people in the world live in malarial areas, about 200 million suffer from malaria every year, and millions are killed by it. Since 1964, China has resumed its research into new anti-malaria drugs, and seeking breakthroughs from Chinese herbal medicines has been the main task of the whole work. However, after sorting out thousands of Chinese herbal medicines, no important discovery was made.

　　从 1969 年开始，屠呦呦开始专心该工作。她整理了历代医籍，编辑了含 640 种药物的《抗疟单验方集》。经过大量的筛选，最后将焦点锁定在青蒿上。她根据东晋名医葛洪《肘后备急方》中"青蒿一握，以水二升渍，绞取汁，尽服之"可治"久疟"的记载，经历了 190 次实验后，终于提取出了对鼠疟、猴疟疟原虫的抑制率达到 100% 的青蒿素。

　　疟疾，一个肆意摧残人类生命健康的恶魔，被一位中国的女性科学家制服了。

　　屠呦呦告诉世界，"青蒿素是人类征服疟疾进程中的一小步，也是中国传统医药献给人类的一份礼物"。

Starting with 1969, Tu Youyou began to concentrate on this research. She sorted out the medical books of the past dynasties and edited the *Kangnüe Dan Yanfang Ji* (*A Collection of Antimalarial Prescriptions*) which lists 640 kinds of drugs. After narrowing down the prescriptions to Artemisia after much assiduous research, she was finally inspired by the descriptions in the *Zhouhou Beiji Fang* (*Handbook of Prescription for Emergencies*) written by Ge Hong, a famous doctor in the Eastern Jin dynasty. The book recorded that malaria can be cured through the prescription of "taking one hold of Artemisia, soaking it into two liters of water, grinding it to extract the juice, and drinking it all". After 190 experiments, Artemisinin was finally extracted, which has a 100% inhibition ratio against malaria parasites in rats and monkeys.

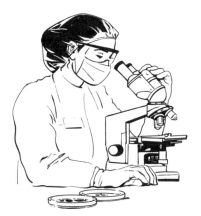

Thus malaria, a monster that had been arbitrarily undermining human life and health, has been completely tamed by a Chinese female scientist.

Tu Youyou has told the world, "the discovery of Artemisinin is only a small step in the process of curing malaria and a gift from Traditional Chinese Medicine to mankind".

第二十二章　走出国门的针灸

针灸是针法和灸法的合称,是中医学的重要组成部分之一,是中华民族文化和科学传统产生的宝贵遗产。2010 年,联合国教科文组织已将"中医针灸"列入"人类非物质文化遗产代表作名录"。

针灸有着悠久的历史,早在公元 6 世纪就传到了朝鲜、日本等国。近年来,随着中外文化交流的不断深入,针灸也随之传到世界各地,每年有近万名留学生来华学习中医药学知识,国际上对针灸的期盼、需求越来越高。

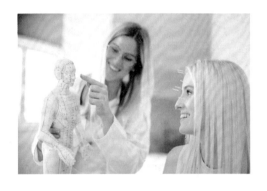

Chapter 22 Acupuncture and Moxibustion Going Abroad

Acupuncture is a combination of acupuncture and moxibustion, which is one of the important components of Traditional Chinese Medicine (TCM) and a valuable heritage of the Chinese cultural and scientific traditions. In 2010, "Acupuncture and moxibustion of TCM " was inscribed on the Representative List of the Intangible Cultural Heritage of Humanity by UNESCO.

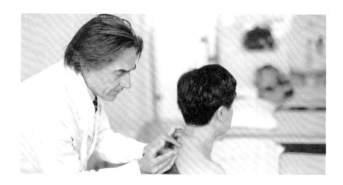

Acupuncture has a long history, spread to Korea, Japan, and other countries as early as the 6th century AD. In recent years, with the deepening of cultural exchanges between China and other countries, acupuncture has been spread to all over the world, and every year nearly 10,000 international students come to China to learn TCM, and the international expectation and demand for acupuncture and moxibustion are rising.

世界上大部分国家或地区都有华人或当地人士开设的中医、针灸诊所。美国登记的职业针灸师有 4 万多人,德国有 3 万名针灸师,墨西哥的针灸师有 5000 多人,澳大利亚有 4500 个针灸、中医师,巴西有针灸师 1.5 万余名,新加坡有中医师 1500 人,中国香港登记的中医、针灸师有 1 万多人,甚至只有两万人口的基里巴斯也有中医诊所。这些数量众多、分布广泛的中医、针灸诊所,为中医药走向世界打下了广泛的基础。

1999 年,瑞士将中医、中药、针灸的费用纳入国民医保。2013 年,匈牙利欧洲第一个实施中医立法,使中医拥有正规的行医许可。比利时已把针灸纳入正规医学。意大利不少医院设有中医门诊部。澳大利亚,70% 的医生会推荐针灸理疗,针灸享有医保补贴。

In most countries or regions of the world, there are Chinese medicine and acupuncture clinics opened by Chinese or local people. There are more than 40,000 registered professional acupuncturists in the United States, 30,000 in Germany, more than 5,000 in Mexico, 4,500 acupuncture and TCM practitioners in Australia, more than 15,000 acupuncturists in Brazil, 1,500 TCM practitioners in Singapore, and more than 10,000 TCM practitioners and acupuncturists registered in Hong Kong, China. Even in Kiribati, which has a small population of only 20,000, there are TCM clinics. These widely distributed TCM and acupuncture clinics have laid a sound foundation for TCM to go global.

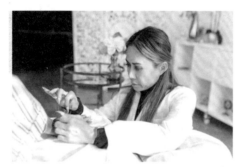

In 1999, Switzerland included the cost of TCM, Chinese materia medica, acupuncture and moxibustion into the national medical insurance. In 2013, Hungary became the first European country to implement legislation on TCM, granting it a formal medical license. Belgium has incorporated acupuncture and moxibustion into regular medicine. Many hospitals in Italy have TCM clinics. In Australia, 70% of doctors will recommend acupuncture and moxibustion physiotherapy, and acupuncture and moxibustion enjoys medical insurance subsidies.

　　法国共有 6 千多名中医从业人员，每年法国境内接受中医诊断治疗约 600 万人次。俄罗斯人看中医已经成为常态，每年有 10 万名俄罗斯患者赴华看中医。美国有 3 万多家中医诊所，每年接受针灸等治疗的人口约 3800 万。

There are over 6,000 TCM practitioners in France, with approximately 6 million people receiving TCM diagnosis and treatment annually. It has become a habit for Russians to see a TCM doctor, with 100,000 Russian patients coming to China for TCM treatment every year. There are more than 30, 000 Chinese medicine clinics in the United States, and about 38 million people receive acupuncture and moxibustion and other Chinese medicine treatments every year.

第二十三章　菲尔普斯的秘密

被誉为"飞鱼"的美国游泳运动员菲尔普斯在奥运比赛中共获得了 23 块金牌，是奥运历史上获得金牌最多的运动员。除了让人叹为观止的成绩外，细心的人会发现菲尔普斯身上总有不少拔罐留下的红印，"奥运冠军偏爱中国拔罐"一时成为媒体的热门话题，中国拔罐被戏称为神秘的"东方力量"。

菲尔普斯接受媒体采访时表示，每次参加完比赛，他都会拔罐，拔火罐能增加灵活性，让酸痛的肌肉能够放松。实际上，拔罐的这一传统中医疗法早就在体育圈成为一种习惯了。运动员们表示，在运动后接受刮痧、拔罐、按摩有助于缓解肌肉酸痛的状况。

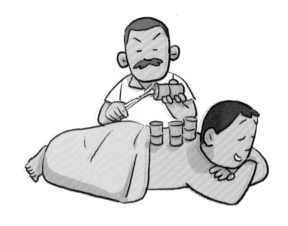

Chapter 23 The Secret of Michael Phelps

Michael Phelps, an American swimmer, who is known as "flying fish", won twenty three Olympic gold medals in total. He is an athlete winning the most gold medals in the Olympic history. In addition to his amazing achievements, people found that Phelps had a lot of red marks on his body left by the cupping therapy. The Olympic champion's preference for Chinese cupping became a hot topic in the media, and Chinese cupping was dubbed as mysterious eastern power.

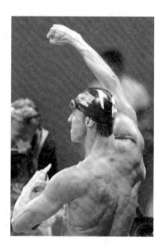

When giving an interview to the media, Phelps said that he would have cupping therapy after each competition, which can increase his flexibility and allow his sore muscles to relax. In fact, cupping therapy, as a Traditional Chinese Medicine (TCM) treatment, has already become a fashion in sports circle. Athletes said that Chinese therapies like scraping, cupping and massage can make their sore muscles relaxing after competitions.

中医拔罐疗法有着悠久的历史，早在西汉时期的帛书《五十二病方》中就有类似火罐疗法的记载。它是以罐为工具，利用燃烧、抽气等方法，形成罐内负压，使之吸附于体表的穴位或患处，形成局部充血或瘀血，而达到活血化瘀、防病治病、强壮身体为目的的一种中医养生方法。具有操作简便、取材容易、见效快、安全可靠的特点，深受群众的喜爱。

Cupping therapy with a long history was first recorded in the silk book (of the Western Han dynasty) named *52 Bing Fang* (*Fifty-two Prescriptions*), which uses cups as a tool, through combustion, pumping and other methods to produce negative pressure in the cupping, so that it can be absorbed on a person's acupoints or infected areas. Thus local congestion or blood stasis appears to achieve the purpose of promoting blood circulation, preventing and treating diseases and strengthening the body. It can be easily and conveniently performed. The cupping materials are easily available too. It is effective, safe and reliable, and is deeply loved by Chinese people.

第二十四章　中医发明人痘接种法

数千年以来，天花作为恶性传染病，造成了大量人口死亡，中国人也深受其害，唐宋以来，天花开始在中国广泛流行。面对肆虐的天花，中医师们，一直探索预防治疗天花的方法，在"以毒攻毒"的思想指导下，中国人发明了人痘接种术。

法国哲学家伏尔泰，这样赞扬人痘接种："我听说一百年来，中国人一直就有这样的习惯；这是被认为全世界最聪明、最讲礼貌的一个民族的伟大先例和榜样。"

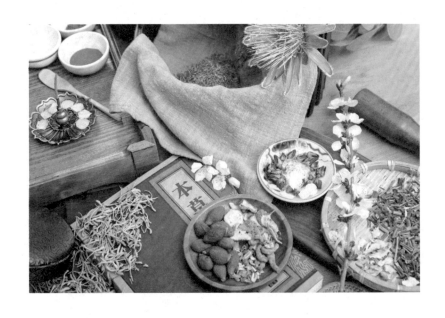

Chapter 24 Variolation in Traditional Chinese Medicine

For thousands of years, smallpox, as a malignant infectious disease, has caused a large number of deaths, and Chinese have also suffered from it too. Since the Tang and Song dynasties, smallpox has been widely spread in China. Faced with its rampant prevalence, traditional Chinese medicine practitioners had been exploring ways to prevent and treat it. Under the guidance of the idea of "combating poison with poison (or like cures like; fight fire with fire)", the Chinese invented variolation.

Voltaire, the famous French philosopher, praised variolation in this way, "I heard that Chinese people have had this habit for a hundred years already; this is a great precedent and example created by a nation considered to be the most intelligent and polite in the world."

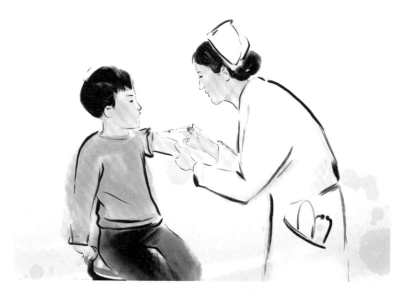

人痘接种，实际上是采用人工的方法，使被接种者感染一次天花。但是，这种早期的种痘术，所使用的都是人身上自然发出的天花的痂，人们把它叫做"时苗"。由于时苗的毒性很大，当中国古代医师们发现由于时苗毒性太大，而造成被接种者死亡之后，他们总结出了两条经验：一是不能用自然之痘作为种苗，也就是不能用时苗接种。二是以使用痘痂为主。以往用痘浆接种的方法被逐渐淘汰。

同时，古人还总结出，人痘接种必须要用"种苗"，而种苗还要经过"养苗""选炼"，使之成为"熟苗"以后才能使用。古人采取的这种通过连续接种和选炼减低痘苗毒性的方法，是合乎现代科学原理的。

人痘接种术的预防效果，不仅使中国人受益，而且引起其他国家的注意与仿效。公元1688年，俄国医生来到北京学习种人痘的方法，不久又从俄国传至土耳其，随即传入英国和欧洲各地。18世纪中叶，人痘接种法已传遍欧亚大陆。人痘接种法的发明，是中国对世界医学的一大贡献。

Variation is actually an artificial method to make the vaccinated person infected with smallpox once. But, an earlier method of vaccination used the scab of smallpox that grew out naturally on human body. People called it "instant vaccine". Because of its great toxicity, ancient TCM practitioners discovered that it might cause the death of the vaccinated. So they summed up two tips: one was that the natural pox could not be used as a vaccine, that is, the instant vaccine could not be used for vaccination. Second, the vaccination of smallpox scab should be widely used. The previous method of vaccination with pox pulp was gradually replaced.

At the same time, ancient Chinese doctors also concluded that human pox vaccination had to use "seedlings", which went through breaking, selecting and refining and became fully ripe. This method was adopted to reduce the toxicity of vaccine through continuous vaccination and selection, which is quite in line with modern scientific principles.

The preventive effect of variolation had not only benefited the Chinese people, but also attracted the attention of other countries that were eager to imitate what had been done in China. In 1688, some Russian doctors came to Beijing to learn the method of variolation, and it soon spread from Russia to Turkey, and then to Britain and all parts of Europe. In the middle of the 18th century, variolation had spread across Europe and Asia. The invention of variolation is surely a great Chinese contribution to world medical development.

第二十五章　中医抗击新冠感染疫情

2020 年以来，以新型冠状病毒感染引起的急性呼吸道传染病逐步席卷全球，造成了严重的人员伤亡。在抗击新冠感染的战斗中，超九成的患者使用了中医药。临床疗效观察，中医药总有效率达 90% 以上。中医药防治新冠感染，成为中国经验的一大亮点。

在中国疫情防控中，经过反复实践，我们形成了以中医药为特色、中西医结合救治患者的新方案。这既是坚持中西医并重的中国卫生健康工作方针，也由中医药具有的独特功效所决定。

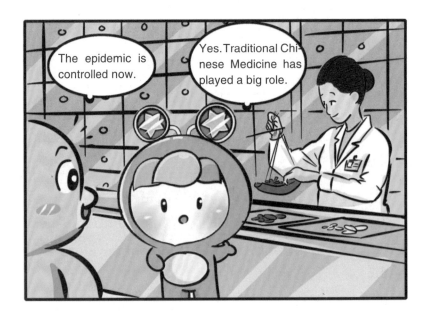

Chapter 25 Traditional Chinese Medicine Fighting the COVID-19 Epidemic

Since the year of 2020, an acute respiratory infectious disease caused by Covid-19 has spread across the world, endangering huge amounts of people. In fighting Covid-19 epidemic, more than 90% of patients took Traditional Chinese Medicine (TCM). Clinical observation showed that the total efficacy rate of TCM was more than 90%. Prevention and treatment of Covid-19 with TCM has become a highlight of China's experience.

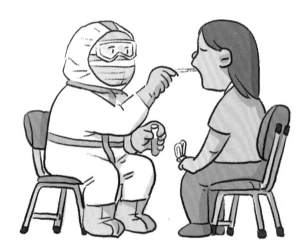

Based on repeated practice, we have promoted a new treatment plan featuring TCM and combining TCM and western medicine to treat patients in epidemic prevention and control. This plan is the Chinese sanitation and health policy which attaches an equal importance to TCM and western medicine, and depends on the unique efficacy of TCM.

在疫情防控时，让发热、留观、密接、疑似这四类人群普服中药，施以标准通治方"中药漫灌"，缩短了症状持续时间，及时截断了疫情的蔓延和扩展势头，从而降低转重率、病亡率。创新了中医药参与社区防护的模式，使防控关口前移至社区。

在重症、康复阶段，采取了中医药辨证论治、一人一方，控制病情恶化发展等，帮助患者更好的康复，减少后遗症。

习近平总书记强调，"中西医结合、中西药并用，是这次疫情防控的一大特点，也是中医药传承精华、守正创新的生动实践"。继承好、发展好、利用好传统医学，让中华文明瑰宝惠及世界，携手应对全球公共卫生挑战，就能为人类健康贡献更多中国智慧和中国力量。

During the period of epidemic prevention and control, four groups of people (patients with fever, patients kept in the hospital for observation, close contacts and suspected cases) took Chinese herbal medicine and were treated with conventional standard method called "TCM flood irrigation", which shortened the symptom duration and timely cut off the spread of epidemic. Therefore the rate of worsening and mortality reduced. We initially promoted the mode of incorporating TCM into community epidemic prevention and control, making the prevention and control front transfer to the community.

During the severe and recovery period, patients were treated with TCM syndrome differentiation with an unique therapy for each person to prevent diseases from worsening, which helped patients get better recovery and reduce the possibility of sequela.

President Xi Jinping of the Communist Party of China emphasized, "one of characteristics in fighting Covid-19 is to combine TCM and western medicine, which is a vivid practice of preserving the essence of TCM, upholding fundamental principles and breaking new grounds". We should inherit, develop and make good use of TCM, letting this gem of Chinese civilization benefit the whole world. When China and other countries work together to meet the challenges faced by global public health, we will contribute our more Chinese wisdom and strength to the improvement of human health.

　　中医药学，是一代代中华民族的行医者在与疾病的不懈斗争中不断探索、逐渐形成的科学认识，是几千年沉淀下来的中国文化精髓。一把草药、一根银针，保佑着中华民族的繁衍昌盛。抗疫战场上，古老的中医焕发着新的生命力，成为抗击疫情的利器。抗击新冠感染疫情的事件再次充分证明，中医药以前是、现在是、未来仍然是人类与瘟疫斗争的重要武器。

TCM is the scientific cognition which has gradually taken its shape in the process of generations of Chinese medical practitioners perversely fighting and exploring diseases, and also the essence of Chinese culture passed down through thousands of years. A hold of herbs and an acupuncture needle guarantee the multiplying and prosperity of the Chinese nation. In the battlefield of fighting Covid-19, ancient TCM is glowing with new vitality and serves as a powerful tool to fight the epidemic. The fact of fighting Covid-19 fully demonstrates one more time that TCM used to be, is and will be a powerful tool to combat the plague.